Self-assessment picture tests
Operative Dentistry

John Glyn Jones
BDS(Lond), PhD(B'ham), LDS,
RCS(Eng), FDS

**Senior Lecturer in
Restorative Dentistry**
University of Leeds
School of Dentistry
UK

**Honorary Consultant in
Restorative Dentistry**
United Leeds Teaching Hospitals NHS Trust
UK

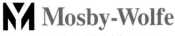 Mosby-Wolfe
London Philadelphia St Louis
Sydney Tokyo

Publisher:	**Jill Northcott**
Development Editor:	**Gillian Harris**
Production:	**Cathy Martin**
Cover Design:	**Greg Smith**

PREFACE

The aim of this book is to give readers an opportunity to test their knowledge in the field of operative dentistry. A wide range of material is presented, some in association with a clinical illustration, others as a simple question. The answers are informative and, it is hoped, go further than just providing the response to the question. By this means the student, whether undergraduate or postgraduate, is provided with an aid to learning. The questions and answers have been provided by a number of experienced clinicians and teachers and, although the main emphasis is on operative dentistry, there is, as could be expected, a slight overlap with the other disciplines comprising restorative dentistry, i.e. endodontics, periodontology and prosthodontics. The questions, which are anonymous, are presented in random order and encompass not only clinical subject matter but also dental materials and related laboratory procedures. Appreciation must be expressed to the contributors who have provided not only the questions and illustrations but also the carefully considered answers. It is hoped that the book will be found of value.

ACKNOWLEDGEMENTS

A number of illustrations have previously been published elsewhere and the Editor is grateful to the publishers of the various journals and books for their ready willingness for them to be reproduced.

Agreement to use *Figure 138* has been given by Dr W.M. Tay. This picture originally appeared in his book *Resin Bonded Bridges* and appreciation is expressed to him and the publishers, Martin Dunitz.

Figure 180 was first used by Dr J. Glyn Jones in *The Dentition and Dental Care* published by Heinemann in 1990, and permission to reproduce it has kindly been given by the editor, Professor R.J. Elderton.

Churchill Livingstone have agreed that *Figures 17, 31, 46, 72* and *134* could be reproduced from *Conservative Dentistry—An integrated approach,* edited by P.H. Jacobsen, and also for *Figure 150*, from *General Dental Treatment, Vol. 2*, edited by Dr W.M. Tay, to be used.

Figures 68, 73, 86, 117 and *146* have previously been used by J.R. Grundy and J. Glyn Jones in their book *A Colour Atlas of Clinical Operative Dentistry, Crowns & Bridges* published by Wolfe Publishing Ltd.

Dental Update has given approval to use *Figure 144*, previously published in a case report in 1983, as has A.E. Morgan for *Figures 123* and *183*, which originally appeared in *Restorative Dentistry*.

Appreciation should finally be recorded to Mr Michael Manogue, Lecturer in Restorative Dentistry, The University of Leeds School of Dentistry, for reading the completed manuscript.

LIST OF CONTRIBUTORS

J. Glyn Jones BDS, PhD, FDSRCS, Senior Lecturer in Restorative Dentistry, The University of Leeds School of Dentistry, Honorary Consultant in Restorative Dentistry, United Leeds Teaching Hospitals NHS Trust.

J.R. Grundy BDS, LDS, MDS, Formerly Senior Lecturer and Tutor in Conservation Techniques, The University of Birmingham School of Dentistry, Consultant Dental Surgeon, Birmingham Area Health Authority (Teaching).

P.H. Jacobsen MDS, FDSRCS, Reader in Restorative Dentistry, University of Wales College of Medicine, Cardiff, Honorary Consultant in Restorative Dentistry, South Glamorgan Health Authority.

E.A.M. Kidd BDS, PhD, FDSRCS, Professor of Cariology, University of London, Honorary Consultant in Restorative Dentistry, United Medical and Dental Schools of Guy's and St Thomas's Hospitals.

L.H. Mair BDS, PhD, Lecturer, Department of Clinical Dental Sciences, University of Liverpool.

B.R. Nattress BChD, FDSRCS, Lecturer in Restorative Dentistry, The University of Leeds School of Dentistry, Honorary Consultant in Restorative Dentistry, United Leeds Teaching Hospitals NHS Trust.

S.E. Northeast BDS, PhD, FDSRCS, Lecturer in Restorative Dentistry, School of Clinical Dentistry, University of Sheffield.

G.J. Pearson BDS, PhD, LDSRCS, Reader in Biomaterials applied to Dentistry, Institute of Dental Surgery, Honorary Consultant in Restorative Dentistry, Eastman Dental Hospital, London.

J.P. Ralph BDS, DDS, HDD (RCPS), FDSRCS, Consultant in Restorative Dentistry, United Leeds Teaching Hospitals NHS Trust.

A.C. Shortall DDS, BDS, FDSRCPS, FFDRCSI, Senior Lecturer in Conservative Dentistry, The University of Birmingham School of Dentistry, Honorary Consultant in Restorative Dentistry, South Birmingham Area Health Authority (Teaching).

B.G.N. Smith BDS, MSc, PhD, FDSRCS, Professor of Conservative Dentistry, University of London, Honorary Consultant in Restorative Dentistry, United Medical and Dental Schools of Guy's and St Thomas's Hospitals.

A.W.G. Walls BDS, PhD, FDSRCS, Professor of Restorative Dentistry, Dental School, University of Newcastle upon Tyne, Honorary Consultant in Restorative Dentistry, Royal Victoria Infirmary and Associated Hospitals NHS Trust.

J.M. Whitworth BChD, PhD, FDSRCS, Lecturer in Operative Dentistry, Dental School, University of Newcastle upon Tyne.

C.C. Youngson BDS, FDSRCS, DRDRCS, Lecturer in Restorative Dentistry, The University of Leeds School of Dentistry.

1 The restoration in the lower first molar shown in *Figure 1* is a high-copper amalgam, while that in the second molar is a low-copper material. Both restorations are 3 years old.
(a) What is the main difference in the constituents of the two materials?
(b) What should be the clinical advantage of the high-copper system?
(c) Outline the difference between the setting reaction of the two types of amalgam.
(d) Is the term non-γ_2 appropriate for all high-copper materials?
(e) Describe the two types of high-copper amalgam currently available.

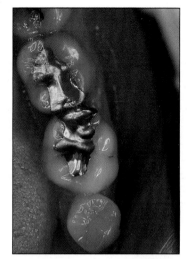

Figure 1

2 The lower premolars and molars in *Figure 2* are of an 18-year-old who has visited your surgery for the first time requesting a checkup.
(a) Do you think caries is present?
(b) How should you examine the teeth?
(c) What special tests might help in the diagnosis?
(d) Why has rubber dam been placed?

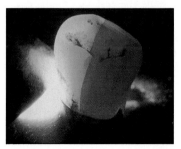

Figure 2

3 (a) Name the investigation that is being undertaken on the isolated lower first pre-molar shown in *Figure 3*.
(b) Describe the various diagnostic situations in which this method of investigation might be useful.

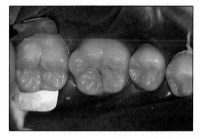

Figure 3

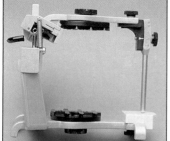

Figure 4

4 (a) Name the type of articulator illustrated in *Figure 4*?
(b) Give the two main uses of the instrument?
(c) What are its limitations in reproducing the function of the patient?

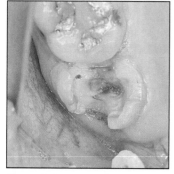

Figure 5

5 During cavity preparation of a symptom-free upper second molar the situation shown in *Figure 5* occurs.
(a) What is your diagnosis and initial treatment?
(b) What steps should be taken subsequently to enable the tooth to be adequately restored?
(c) What do you anticipate will be the final restoration and why?
(d) Following successful restoration what monitoring of the tooth will be required?

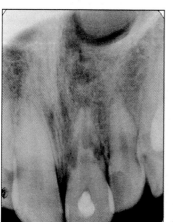

6 (a) Describe the pathology that the radiograph shown in *Figure 6* exhibits.
(b) What is the possible aetiology?
(c) Discuss the short- and long-term management of the condition.

Figure 6

7 (a) What has probably caused this tooth (*Figure 7*) to discolour?
(b) Explain the mechanism by which the discoloration has occurred.

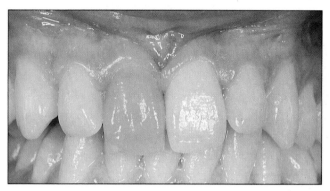

Figure 7

8 A gel has been applied (*Figure 8*) to this fractured ceramic
surface.
(a) Describe the possible active constituents of the gel and
discuss what role they play in the process of repairing ceramic
restorations.
(b) What material should be used for the repair and what other
steps would you take to ensure a satisfactory bond to the ceramic
surface?

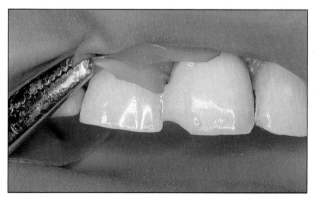

Figure 8

9 Two varieties of light-curing units are shown in *Figure 9* for the polymerisation of photoinitiated composites.
(a) Describe the mechanism involved in the polymerisation process.
(b) Give the advantages and disadvantages of each type of unit.

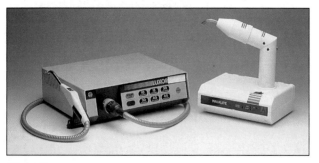

Figure 9

10 (a) What are the effects of age on the salivary flow rates in man?
(b) Outline other factors which will influence salivary function and suggest the effects of reduced flow in the oral cavity.
(c) Describe the rationale behind the use of an artificial saliva. What are the desirable features of a salivary substitute?

11 A demineralised histological section of a tooth (*Figure 10*) shows the floor of a cavity separated from the dental pulp by a thin wall of dentine.
(a) What stain has been used in the preparation of the specimen?
(b) Describe the general condition of the pulpal tissue.
(c) What other points of interest are visible?
(d) What clinical signs and symptoms might be exhibited by a tooth with this pulpal histology?

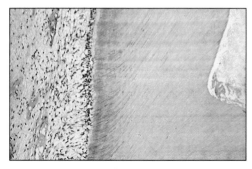

Figure 10

12 (a) Name the finishing lines used in the extracoronal preparation of teeth illustrated in *Figure 11*.
(b) Discuss the types of preparation for which they are indicated and give the advantages and disadvantages of each.

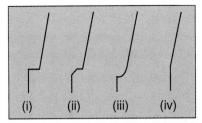

Figure 11

13 An MOD composite resin restoration (*Figure 12*) in the lower first molar has failed.
(a) What features of the restoration justify this statement?
(b) Given that the use of posterior composites is controversial, what guidelines would you consider to be generally acceptable for the use of posterior composites?

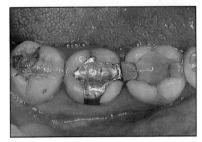

Figure 12

14 The cavity illustrated in *Figure 13* requires a base prior to permanent restoration.
(a) Give the functions of a base material.
(b) What types of material are currently available to fulfil these requirements?
(c) Outline the advantages and disadvantages of each material that you include.

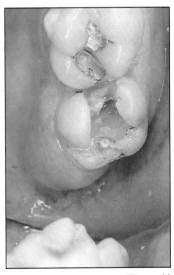

Figure 13

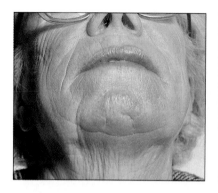

15 A 64-year-old lady returns to your surgery complaining of an itchy face rash (*Figure 14*) that developed after your recent examination.
(a) What may be responsible for this phenomenon?
(b) Indicate the precautions you would take when treating this patient in the future.

Figure 14

16 *Figure 15* is a radiograph of an 18-year-old who has visited your surgery for the first time and requested a checkup.
(a) Name the radiographic view and suggest reasons why it will have been taken.
(b) How would you know which way round to view the film?
(c) Report on the radiograph.
(d) Comment on the appearance of the approximal surfaces between the upper premolars.
(e) What is the radiolucent shadow on the mesial aspect of the upper first molar?

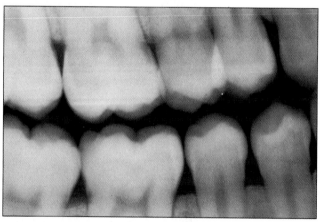

Figure 15

17 Describe how incomplete coronal fractures can be detected.

18 An upper right central incisor (*Figure 16*) has been restored on a number of occasions with a post crown that has repeatedly become dislodged.
(a) What are the most likely causes of the failure?
(b) Before a further attempt to restore the tooth is undertaken what investigations are required?
(c) According to your findings, what would be your treatment plans?

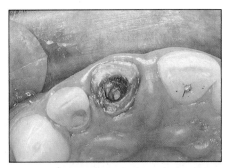

Figure 16

19 (a) What name is given to the red plastic coverings which can be seen (*Figure 17*) on these two teeth?
(b) For what purpose will they be used?
(c) From what can they be constructed and how are they made?

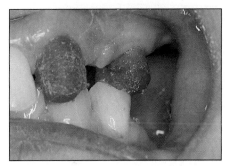

Figure 17

20 The extra-oral lesion illustrated in *Figure 18* has a dental cause.
(a) How would a definitive diagnosis be made of the cause?
(b) How should the condition be treated?

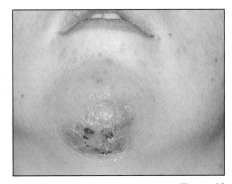

Figure 18

11

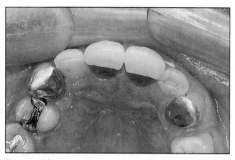

Figure 19

21 The 60-year-old patient, shown in *Figure 19*, works in a high-stress profession and complained of repeated fracture of restorations in his posterior teeth.
(a) Give the likely reason for the failure of the posterior restorations?
(b) How may the gold restorations on the canines alleviate the problem?

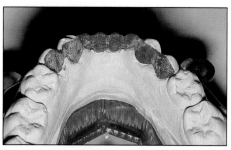

Figure 20

22 An acrylic resin is being used (*Figure 20*) to construct a pattern for casting a long-span minimal preparation bridge.
(a) What problem may result from the use of this technique?
(b) Describe an alternative method that overcomes the problem.
(c) Are there any limitations in using the alternative technique?

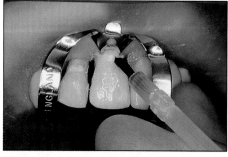

Figure 21

23 *Figure 21* shows the application of a low-viscosity bonding resin to the acid-etched enamel and the glass-ionomer (polyalkenoate) lining of a Class V cavity before restoration with a composite resin. What is the advantage to be gained clinically from using a low-viscosity intermediary resin before composite resin placement?

24 Traditionally, it has been difficult to attach gold alloys (*Figure 22*) to tooth substance using adhesive luting agents.
(a) Describe the techniques that are now available to enable a durable bond to be formed between the fit surface of gold castings and adhesive resins.
(b) What are the advantages of using gold as the contacting surface for restorations opposing natural tissue compared with using either non-precious metals or porcelain?
(c) Having prepared a casting with a gold occlusal surface, describe the surface finish you would ask your technician to prepare prior to cementation.

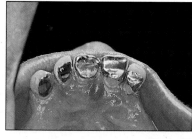

Figure 22

25 The impression shown in *Figure 23* was taken in a condensation silicone elastomer using a two-stage technique.
(a) Is this a suitable impression material to record the detail of a crown preparation?
(b) What are the advantages of a two-stage impression technique?
(c) Are there any disadvantages to this technique and if so what are they?

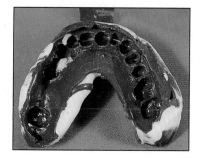

Figure 23

26 The wing of a resin-bonded bridge has been electrolytically etched (*Figure 24*).
(a) Why has this been done?
(b) What other surface treatments of retainer wings can be carried out?
(c) Describe the types of luting materials that are available to cement this type of bridge.

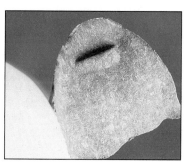

Figure 24

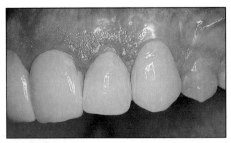

Figure 25

27 (a) Describe the clinical appearance of the gingival margin of the recently restored upper left lateral incisor shown in *Figure 25*.
(b) What may have contributed to the event?
(c) Outline any treatment that is indicated.

28 What are the advantages and disadvantages of zinc phosphate and glass-ionomer (polyalkenoate) luting cements?

29 The restoration in the lower canine shown in *Figure 26* is a glass-ionomer (polyalkenoate) cement from which the matrix has just been removed.
(a) What is the next stage in the clinical procedure and why is it important?
(b) How is the stage best achieved and what options could be considered?
(c) When would you propose finishing the restoration?

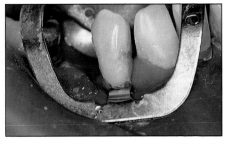

Figure 26

(d) What is the main advantage of glass-ionomer cements over other filling materials?
(e) The material illustrated is a Type II aesthetic glass-ionomer. What other types are available and how do they differ?

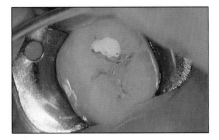

Figure 27

30 (a) What restoration is being carried out in *Figure 27*?
(b) Why has this operative management been chosen?
(c) Why is a rubber dam being used?
(d) Describe, giving the reason, the appearance of the enamel.
(e) What is the white material in the base of the cavity?

31 *Figure 28* shows the maxillary first permanent molar of a 43-year-old female who is complaining of pain on biting. Further examination reveals that the tooth has a complete vertical fracture running mesio-distally, cleanly dividing the palatal from the buccal roots. The three roots are free from further fracture and have good bony support.

Outline possible approaches for the management of this tooth, giving the advantages and disadvantages of each treatment option.

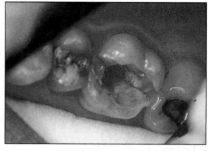

Figure 28

32 The addition-cure polyvinyl-siloxane impression material shown in *Figure 29* is being incorrectly mixed.
(a) What error is being committed?
(b) Discuss the effect this would have on the material?
(c) Describe other methods of mixing that would overcome this problem?

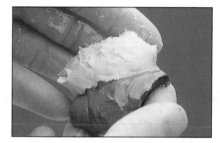

Figure 29

33 Three years previously, the 30-year-old female patient shown in *Figure 30* had her proclined upper incisors restored (repositioned) by means of post crowns. She now complains that the teeth are moving and spaces are developing between them.
(a) How would you investigate the complaint?
(b) What are the likely reasons for tooth movement?
(c) How can the situation be rectified?

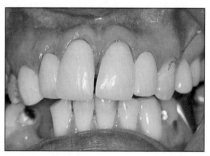

Figure 30

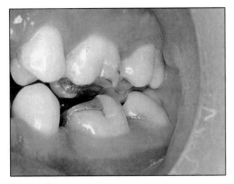

Figure 31

34 This photograph of the left side of the mouth (*Figure 31*) has been taken when the patient moved the mandible to the right.
(a) Name the tooth contact that is shown.
(b) Discuss its significance.

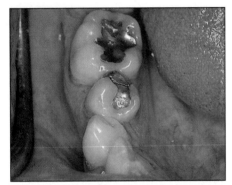

Figure 32

35 The amalgam restoration in the premolar tooth shown in *Figure 32* has failed.
(a) Why is the restoration unsatisfactory?
(b) What are the possible causes for the failure?
(c) How might the occurrence be prevented in the replacement restoration?

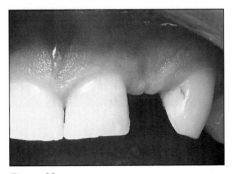

Figure 33

36 A resin-bonded bridge has failed, leaving an edentulous space (*Figure 33*). Recurrent caries mesially on the upper left canine requires treatment before reconstructing the bridge. How would you replace this restoration to obtain the best possible bond between the restoration and the replacement bridge?

37 A patient complains of the discoloured appearance of the upper central incisors (*Figure 34*), which had been root-filled some years previously. The patient has noticed an increase in the discoloration over the past 12–18 months. Clinical examination reveals that the crowns of the teeth are intact apart from palatal amalgam restorations, which have been used to restore the access cavities.

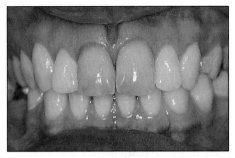

Figure 34

(a) What possible options are there for restoring the upper central incisor teeth?
(b) Outline the advantages and disadvantages of each method.

38 One of your regular 45-year-old patients attends your surgery for a 1-year review appointment and five new root-surface carious lesions (*Figure 35*) are identified.
(a) Which physical characteristics are the most reliable predictors of disease activity in such cases?
(b) What aetiological factors have probably contributed to the present situation?

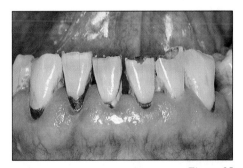

Figure 35

(c) How would you manage this case clinically and what advice would you give the patient?
(d) Is the prevalence of root-surface caries influenced by the fluoridation of the water supply?

39 A 27-year-old patient attends the hospital following a skiing accident. The upper left canine (*Figure 36*) has been traumatised and fractured diagonally in the longitudinal plane from buccal to palatal through the pulp. The palatal margin is approximately 3 mm below the gingival margin.

Both upper and lower arches are otherwise intact.

(a) Outline the initial treatment that you would undertake.
(b) What methods are available for exposing the palatal margin?
(c) Why is it necessary to expose this sub-gingival margin?

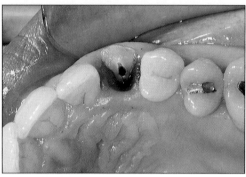

Figure 36

40 (a) Discuss the possible aetiology that could have led to the appearance (*Figure 37*) of these lower second molars.
(b) What problems might you encounter in attempting to restore these teeth?
(c) Outline, with reasons, the treatment you would provide?

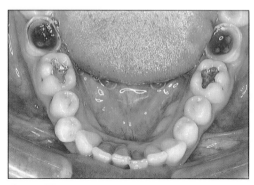

Figure 37

41 The upper left first pre-molar tooth has been restored with a porcelain inlay (*Figure 38*) manufactured at the chairside by a CAD/CAM technique.
(a) What does CAD/CAM stand for?
(b) What are the current limitations of available CAD/CAM techniques?

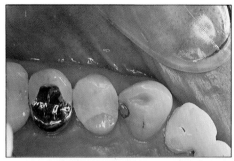

Figure 38

42 A scanning electron micrograph (*Figure 39*) shows a low-copper amalgam restoration after 3 years of clinical service.
(a) What has happened at the margin?
(b) Describe why the situation has occurred.
(c) Should the restoration be replaced? Give your reasons.
(d) Regardless of the type of amalgam used, which clinical procedure minimises the phenomenon?

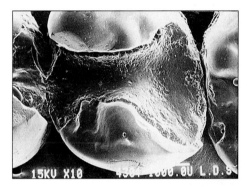

Figure 39

43 *Figure 40* shows a large Class IV cavity in an elderly patient. The lining is a light-cured glass-ionomer.
(a) Which type of material should be used for the final restoration of this tooth?
(b) How will the material be retained?
(c) Is a lining absolutely necessary in this case? What would be the advantages of using a glass-ionomer lining?
(d) What is the clinical advantage of using light-cured glass-ionomer linings?

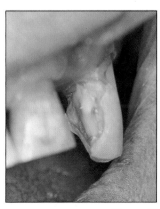

Figure 40

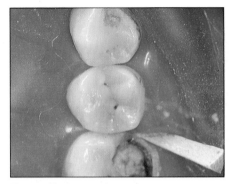

Figure 41

44 (a) Describe the occlusal surface of the lower second premolar (*Figure 41*) in this 20-year-old patient.
(b) What special tests would you undertake before treating the tooth?

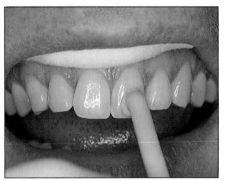

Figure 42

45 (a) What is the test (*Figure 42*) being undertaken on this maxillary left central incisor?
(b) How would you expect this tooth to respond if its pulp was irreversibly inflamed?

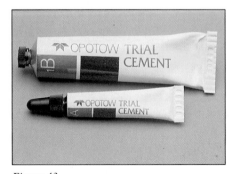

Figure 43

46 (a) For what is the material shown in *Figure 43* used?
(b) Describe its advantages over others which may be used in this situation?

47 A 40-year-old male patient attends, requesting that his anterior teeth be crowned because they are 'wearing away' (*Figures 44* and *45*).
(a) What investigations are required in order that a diagnosis can be made and a treatment plan formulated?
(b) If the anterior teeth are to be crowned, what additional treatment will be necessary to ensure that the crowns are satisfactory?

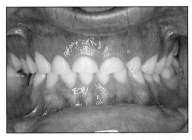

Figure 44   Figure 45

48 (a) Name the appliance that is illustrated in *Figure 46*.
(b) Discuss its clinical application.

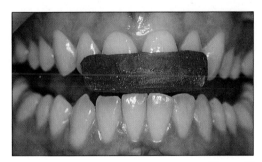

Figure 46

49 (a) What is the likely cause for the appearance of the teeth shown in *Figure 47*?
(b) Is it possible to determine at what age the condition developed and if so, when?
(c) What treatment options are available?

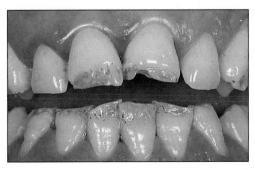

Figure 47

50 The post crown illustrated in *Figure 48* has been recemented on three previous occasions. The patient does not want the crown remade and requests that it be recemented again. A stage in the preparation of the restoration for recementing is shown in *Figure 49*.
(a) Outline the possible causes for the repeated failure of this restoration.
(b) What precautions are essential when recementing a dislodged crown?
(c) How is the fitting surface being treated in this case?
(d) What is the purpose of the treatment?

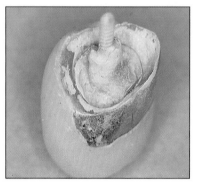

Figure 48

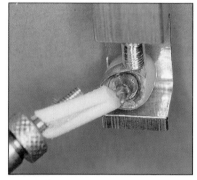

Figure 49

51 The palatal cusp of an upper first premolar (*Figure 50*) has fractured and been lost.
(a) Describe the sequence of events that may have led to this occurrence.
(b) What symptoms may the patient have experienced?
(c) How may the tooth be restored?

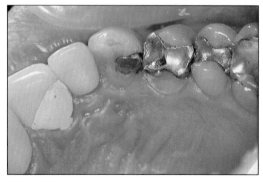

Figure 50

52 You have just placed glass-ionomer (polyalkenoate) restorations in the upper right canine and premolars (*Figure 51*). The patient is unhappy with the appearance.
(a) What is the problem?
(b) How would you manage the situation?
(c) How should a freshly placed glass-ionomer restoration be finished?

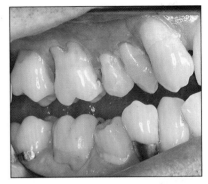

Figure 51

53 The bridge shown in *Figure 52* has been constructed from ceramic fused to metal.
(a) Upon what criteria do you base a decision to use this combination of materials?
(b) What determines whether ceramic or metal is used on the occlusal surfaces of posterior teeth?
(c) What would be the cement of choice for the retention of these crowns?
(d) Describe the necessary differences in preparation of teeth to receive either metal–ceramic crowns, all-metal or all-porcelain crowns.

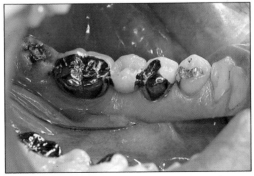

Figure 52

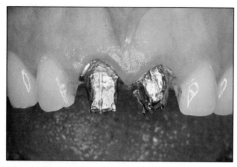

Figure 53

54 The crowns on the upper central incisors were sectioned and removed because of poor aesthetics (*Figure 53*).
(a) What can be seen covering the preparations?
(b) Why is this an unusual finding?
(c) In which type of porcelain crown might you expect to find a similar material as an integral part of the crown?
(d) Why will it have been used?

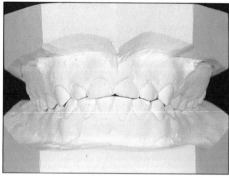

Figure 54

55 *Figure 54* shows the study casts for a 16-year-old patient with bulimia nervosa.
(a) What do you observe and indicate what you would expect to find if you looked at the palatal surfaces of the upper incisor teeth?
(b) Of what is the patient likely to complain?
(c) Describe treatment options that you can offer.

56 Describe the factors which dictate the position of gingival margins for:
(a) Amalgam restorations.
(b) Composite restorations.
(c) Extracoronal restorations.

57 An anterior composite restoration (*Figure 55*) has recurrent caries after 4 years of clinical service.
(a) Why has the restoration failed at this site?
(b) How would you manage the case?
(c) If the whole restoration needed replacement, how would you minimise the chances of recurrent failure?

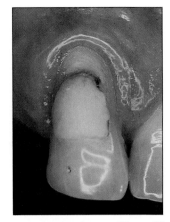

Figure 55

58 Access has been gained (*Figure 56*) to a large carious cavity on the occlusal aspect of a symptom-less and vital lower second premolar in a 20-year-old patient. (Note that *Figure 41* shows the clinical appearance of the tooth before cavity preparation was started.)
(a) Why is the dentist using rubber dam?
(b) Having gained access to the caries, what will be the next stage?
(c) How should caries be removed from over the pulp?
(d) How should the tooth be treated if a carious exposure is found?

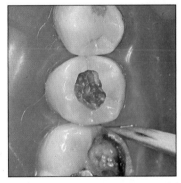

Figure 56

59 (a) What are the various radiographic views that might be needed to formulate a treatment plan that encompasses all aspects of restorative dentistry?
(b) What information would you hope to gain from these films?

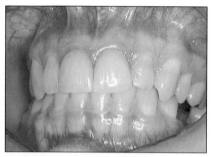

Figure 57

60 A 20-year-old woman has attended, complaining of poor aesthetics following the cementation of two porcelain veneers (*Figure 57*) on the central incisors 2 months ago.
(a) What is the reason for the appearance?
(b) Describe the steps that would be required to produce acceptable aesthetics?

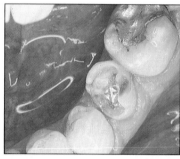

Figure 58

61 (a) What means of providing additional retention is being used in the restoration of the lower premolar shown in *Figure 58*?
(b) What are the potential difficulties that might be encountered with the use of such a technique?
(c) Suggest other methods which could be considered to aid restoration of such a tooth.

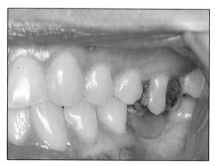

Figure 59

62 (a) Describe the occlusal arrangement illustrated in *Figure 59*.
(b) Outline your treatment plan to provide a prosthesis to replace the single missing lower molar.
(c) What are the possible consequences of leaving such a condition unrestored?

63 *Figure 60* shows a radiograph of a 20-year-old patient who was attending your surgery for the first time.
(a) What is the radiographic view and why has it been taken?
(b) Comment on the radiographic appearance of the lower first molar and describe how this will effect your management of the tooth.
(c) Comment on the radiographic appearance of the lower second

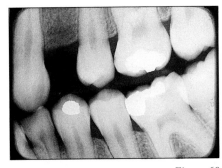

Figure 60

premolar and on your management of the tooth.
(d) Comment on the radiographic appearance of the upper first molar and discuss your management of the tooth.

64 *Figure 61* shows a longitudinal section through an MOD direct composite restoration, bonded to the tooth using enamel etching and a dentine bonding system. Prior to sectioning, the tooth was immersed in methylene blue dye for 24 h.
(a) What is the significance of the stained area of dentine either side of the axiogingival line angle on the left of the picture?
(b) What are the likely causes for this occurrence?
(c) How can they be minimised?

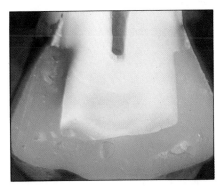

Figure 61

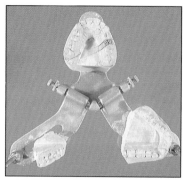

Figure 62

65 *Figure 62* shows the three-arm configuration of a twin-stage occluder articulator (Hanau) with mounted casts and FGP functional index opposing the occlusal surface of a full veneer crown restoration of a maxillary premolar.
(a) What are the reasons for using this technique and how does it minimise the need for intra-oral adjustments of restorations?
(b) Give the main clinical requirements for the successful use of the technique.

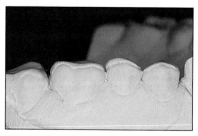

Figure 63

66 The teeth shown in *Figure 63* have been restored by means of partial coverage restorations.
(a) Describe the appearance of the teeth.
(b) How would you attempt to identify the cause of the condition?
(c) Discuss the differential diagnosis and indicate the most likely cause.
(d) Discuss the suitability of providing this type of restoration in this situation.

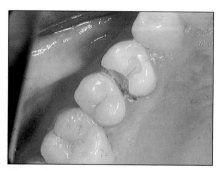

Figure 64

67 An upper first premolar (*Figure 64*) has been prepared to receive an amalgam restoration.
(a) What faults can be identified in the cavity preparation?
(b) Discuss how these would lead to a failure of the restoration if the cavity remains unmodified.

68 How has the under-
standing of the behaviour
of carious lesions altered
the role of the instrument
shown in *Figure 65* in
caries diagnosis in recent
years?

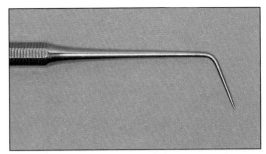

Figure 65

69 You have decided to provide a fixed bridge prosthesis, replacing the upper left
second premolar for a patient with the first premolar and molar as the abutment
teeth. The anterior retainer is a metal–ceramic crown, while that for the distal tooth
is a gold alloy partial veneer crown. The pontic is of a modified ridge lap design,
having a metal occlusal surface and a porcelain buccal veneer. At try-in, the bridge
fails to seat fully on the anterior abutment. Outline possible reasons for this and the
approach you would adopt to deal with the occurrence.

70 (a) Suggest the possible
causes for the development
of a midline diastema, such
as that shown in *Figure 66*.
(b) How could you demon-
strate to the patient how various non-orthodontic options
could alter the appearance
prior to the commencement
of operative treatment?
(c) Why is it important to
demonstrate to patients what
the effect of treatment might
be?

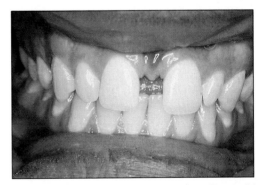

Figure 66

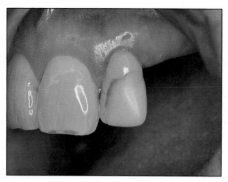

Figure 67

71 (a) What is the likely cause of the marginal stain associated with the anterior composite shown in *Figure 67* that has been in place for 6 years?
(b) How can it be prevented from occurring?
(c) What are the two main types of composite available today?
(d) Describe the major difference in their clinical appearance.
(e) Identify the type illustrated.

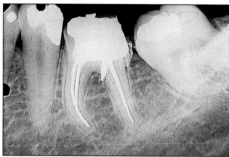

Figure 68

72 (a) What faulty treatment is demonstrated by the radiograph shown in *Figure 68*?
(b) Outline factors which might have contributed to the occurrence?
(c) Suggest possible treatment options.

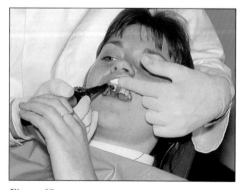

Figure 69

73 (a) What is the procedure that the clinician in *Figure 69* is undertaking?
(b) Give reasons for:
• The paste on the labial surface of the tooth.
• Interproximal placement of rubber dam.
• Patient contact with the appliance.

74 *Figure 70* shows a bridge that has been made to replace the missing lateral incisor using a previously unrestored vital central and root-filled, post/cored canine.
(a) Name the type of bridge?
(b) Discuss the rationale for its use in this case?
(c) What alternative designs could have been considered?

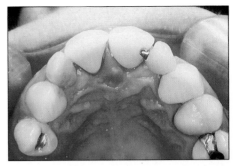

Figure 70

75 A post crown has been lost from an upper right central incisor (*Figure 71*).
(a) Why has the restoration failed?
(b) What methods are available to re-establish the post hole?
(c) If these techniques fail, what alternative method of core construction is possible?

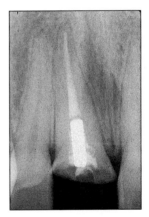

Figure 71

76 (a) What clinical errors or deficiencies can be identified in *Figure 72*?
(b) Discuss their possible consequences.

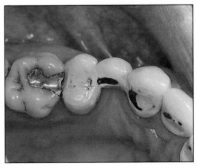

Figure 72

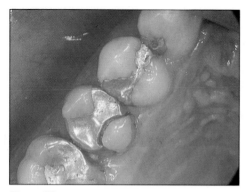

Figure 73

77 (a) What has happened to the upper second premolar shown in *Figure 73*, and why?
(b) How could it have been prevented?
(c) What treatment is now indicated?

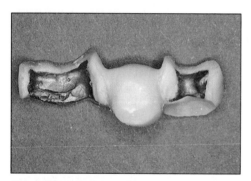

Figure 74

78 The bridge illustrated in *Figure 74* is of an unorthodox design.
(a) Why is it unorthodox?
(b) Upon what does the success of this design depend?
(c) Suggest alternative designs and give the reasons for your choice.

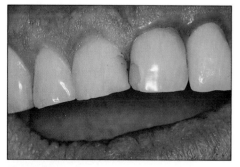

Figure 75

79 The mesial composite resin restorations in the upper central incisors (*Figure 75*) have been in place for 8 years.
(a) Describe the appearance of the fillings.
(b) Suggest possible reasons for the occurrence.
(c) Indicate ways of improving the situation.

80 A patient (*Figure 76*) gives a history of a blow to the face while playing football some 2 years previously.
(a) What is the most likely cause of the discoloration of the upper right central incisor?
(b) What investigations would you undertake to confirm your diagnosis?
(c) Describe your proposed treatment for the patient, indicating the complications that you might anticipate.

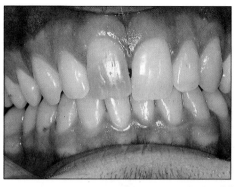

Figure 76

81 (a) What procedure is being carried out on the upper premolar shown in *Figure 77*?
(b) Why is it being undertaken?
(c) Describe other methods which could be utilised to achieve the same result, giving the advantages and disadvantages of each technique.

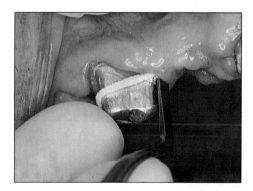

Figure 77

82 A routine radiographic examination reveals an unusual finding (*Figure 78*).
(a) Describe the radiographic appearance of the upper left first molar.
(b) Suggest explanations for its occurrence.
(c) What are the treatment options and what would be the probable sequelae if the condition was left?

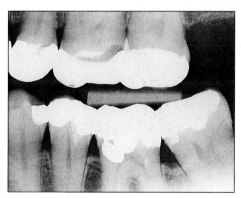

Figure 78

83 (a) What are the requirements of a provisional crown-and-bridge material?
(b) How do the currently available resin-based materials perform against these requirements?
(c) What would be the most appropriate material(s) for provisional crown-and-bridge construction where occlusal considerations are paramount?

84 The model shown in *Figure 79* was cast from an addition-cured silicone impression, immediately following its removal from the mouth.
(a) What has led to this appearance?
(b) How might it effect any cast restoration constructed on the model?
(c) Describe how the impression should have been handled in order to avoid such an occurrence.

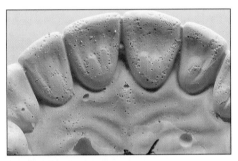

Figure 79

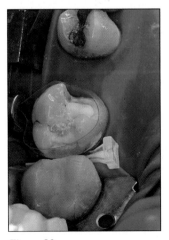

85 A tooth (*Figure 80*) is about to be restored with a posterior composite.
(a) Why is it difficult to attain a good marginal bond at the cervical margin?
(b) Describe clinical procedures you would adopt to minimise the problem.
(c) How does the refractive wedge help?

Figure 80

86 A 23-year-old patient attends your surgery because they have bleeding gums (*Figure 81*).
(a) Describe the appearance of the gums.
(b) What do you think will happen when you run a blunt periodontal probe along the gingival margins?
(c) Comment on the appearance of the enamel around the gum margins.
(d) How will you begin to manage the conditions?

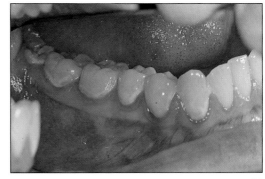

Figure 81

87 What are the possible advantages to be gained by the routine use of the technique shown in *Figure 82* for operative dentistry procedures?

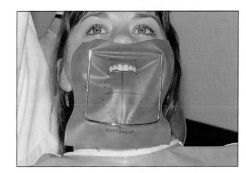

Figure 82

88 In *Figure 83* why has the tooth substance been retained prior to restoration with a cermet core?

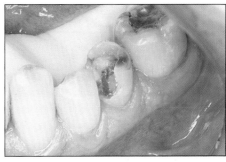

Figure 83

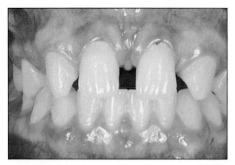

Figure 84

89 A 16-year-old girl is worried about the appearance of her upper anterior teeth (*Figure 84*).
(a) What treatment options are available and how could these be undertaken?
(b) At what age should each treatment be commenced?

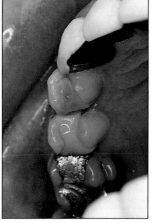

Figure 85

90 (a) List the faults that can be identified in relation to the composite restorations in the two upper premolars shown in *Figure 85*.
(b) What are the likely causes of the deficiencies?

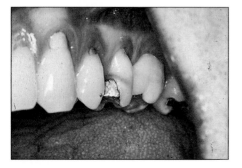

91 (a) How can the light and dark bands (*Figure 86*) around the amalgam filling in this upper first premolar be explained?
(b) What further investigations and treatment are indicated?

Figure 86

92 *Figure 87* illustrates a defect at the gingival margin of a laminate veneer on the upper left canine.
(a) What material has been used to construct the veneer and why has the defect occurred?
(b) How can the problem be avoided?
(c) Is the problem likely to occur with other types of veneer material?
(d) How could you repair or mask the defect?

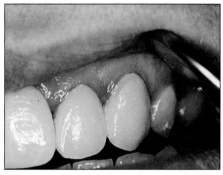

Figure 87

93 (a) What stage of cavity preparation is being undertaken in *Figure 88*?
(b) If a composite resin restoration were to be planned, describe what other requirements for successful restoration retention would be necessary if no additional 'macroscopic' mechanical retention is planned for the cavity preparation.

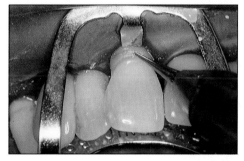

Figure 88

94 (a) What are the differences in the pattern of polymerisation between self-cured and visible-light activated composite resins?
(b) How do these differences influence the effects of polymerisation shrinkage upon tooth restoration?
(c) What are the detrimental effects of polymerisation contraction, and how may they be overcome?

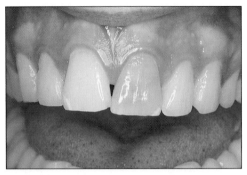

Figure 89

95 (a) What simple and relatively non-destructive method could be employed to improve the dark appearance of an adequately root-filled and symptom-free upper incisor (*Figure 89*), which has, other than the access cavity, an intact crown?
(b) Outline the stages in the technique.
(c) What complications may occur?

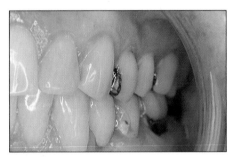

Figure 90

96 This patient complains about the appearance of the upper left first premolar (*Figure 90*). Suggest ways by which its appearance could be improved?

97 (a) Which of the following cutting techniques will produce the minimal pulpal injury?
    (i)   Air turbine at 300,000 rev/min with air coolant.
    (ii) Conventional engine at 5000 rev/min with no coolant.
    (iii) Air turbine at 300,000 rev/min with water spray coolant.
(b) What is the first sign in the microscopic appearance of the pulp of careless cavity preparation?
    (i)   Inflammatory cells in the sub-odontoblastic layer.
    (ii) Displacement of odontoblastic nuclear material into dentinal tubules.
    (iii) Hyperaemia.
    (iv) Hydropic degeneration of pulpal cells.
(c) Early pulpal inflammation is associated with pain in which of the following circumstances?
    (i)   With hot and cold food.
    (ii) On biting.
    (iii) Only at night-time.
    (iv) Spontaneously.

98 (a) What is revealed by the radiograph shown in *Figure 91*?
(b) What aspects of filling technique would have prevented the failure from occurring?

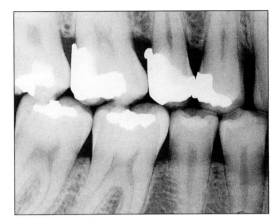

Figure 91

99 A composite inlay (*Figure 92*) is being manufactured by the chairside extra-oral approach.
(a) In this case, what are the advantages and disadvantages of the technique over a direct placement composite?
(b) What are the general advantages of indirect composites (inlays) over direct placement materials?
(c) Which type of material would you use to cement the inlay?

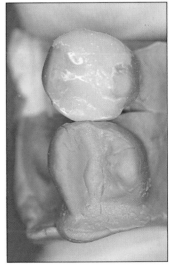

Figure 92

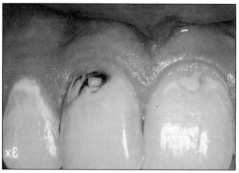
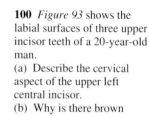

Figure 93

100 *Figure 93* shows the labial surfaces of three upper incisor teeth of a 20-year-old man.
(a) Describe the cervical aspect of the upper left central incisor.
(b) Why is there brown staining on the labial aspect of the lateral incisor?
(c) Would you, giving your reasons, replace the filling on the labial aspect of the upper right central incisor?

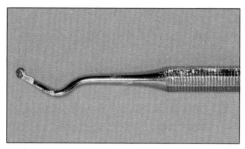
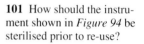

Figure 94

101 How should the instrument shown in *Figure 94* be sterilised prior to re-use?

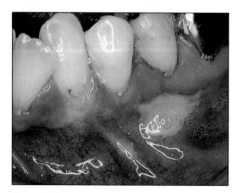

Figure 95

102 The ulcer shown in *Figure 95* has appeared the day following the administration of a mental block given to allow a lower first premolar to be restored with composite resin.
(a) Why might the ulcer have developed?
(b) What steps should have been taken to prevent its occurrence?
(c) Give the constituents of a local anaesthetic cartridge and indicate the reasons for their inclusion.

103 Having worn a simple acrylic partial denture for a number of years a 40-year-old patient requests replacement of his missing upper incisors (*Figure 96*) with a fixed bridge. He has good oral hygiene and a well-maintained mouth.

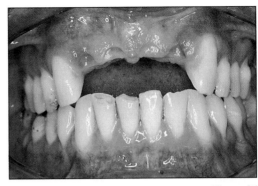

Figure 96

(a) What potential difficulties can be foreseen if such treatment was to be attempted?
(b) What alternative treatment options should be discussed with the patient?
(c) If fixed bridgework were undertaken, suggest a suitable design for this clinical situation.

104 This patient is concerned about the appearance of her anterior teeth (*Figure 97*). Suggest ways in which the aesthetics might be improved.

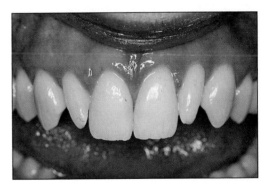

Figure 97

105 Describe how the design, preparation and completion of dental restorations may affect the progress of dental disease.

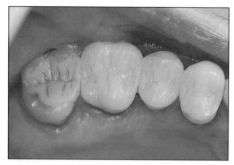

Figure 98

106 The teeth shown in *Figure 98* have been restored with ceramic inlays and onlays.
(a) How are the restorations retained in the preparations?
(b) Why do the restorations blend well with the remaining tooth structure?
(c) What long-term problems may be observed when the restorations are reviewed?

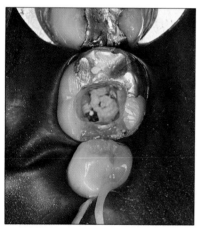

Figure 99

107 A first lower molar tooth has been root-filled and the access cavity (*Figure 99*) requires restoration before the tooth can be crowned. The remaining disto-occluso-lingual part of the existing amalgam restoration is sound and effectively pin-retained.
(a) What techniques are available for core build-up prior to crown preparation?
(b) Indicate, with reasons, the approach that you would adopt in this instance.

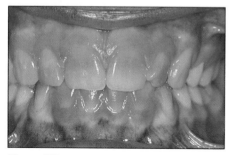

Figure 100

108 (a) What may have been responsible for the discoloration of these teeth (*Figure 100*) in a 16-year-old girl?
(b) Describe the treatment options that are available for the management of the discoloration.
(c) Upon what would you base your preferred treatment?

109 A patient attends your surgery complaining about a broken lower back tooth (*Figure 101*). A vitality test indicates that it is vital and the periapical radiograph shows no apical changes.
(a) Describe your initial treatment.
(b) Would auxiliary means of retaining the restoration be indicated and, if so, what would you propose using?
(c) Indicate, with reasons, your long-term treatment for the tooth.

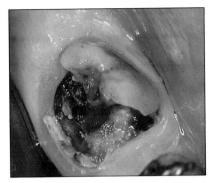

Figure 101

110 This resin-bonded bridge (*Figure 102*) became detached at the distal wing 1 week following cementation.
(a) List the design faults which may have contributed to the failure.
(b) What are the key features of tooth preparation for resin-bonded bridges?
(c) Describe what features should be checked at the try-in stage.

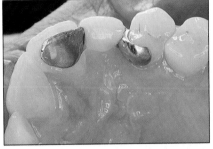

Figure 102

111 Composite restorations have been placed in several of the upper teeth. The restorations in the upper right lateral and canine teeth (*Figure 103*) show a white line around the neck. What is the likely cause of this?

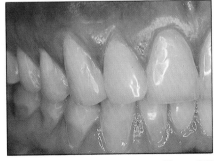

Figure 103

112 (a) What types of elastomeric impression materials are available to record details of preparations in order that a bridge can be constructed?
(b) Describe their major advantages and disadvantages.

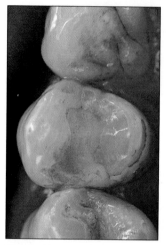

Figure 104

113 While looking at the extraction site a few days after the removal of a wisdom tooth a patient became concerned that a new 'white' filling (*Figure 104*) had become discoloured.
(a) Indicate the likely cause of the discoloration.
(b) Why does it occur?
(c) What treatment would you provide?
(d) Discuss the general significance of the effect.

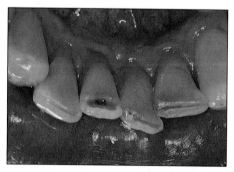

Figure 105

114 A 60-year-old lady (*Figure 105*) has Sjögren's syndrome.
(a) What is Sjögren's syndrome?
(b) What dental complications of the syndrome can be seen in the picture?
(c) How would you decide whether to manage the lesion in the lower right central incisor operatively?

115 You have just recorded an impression (*Figure 106*) of a full-veneer crown preparation in an addition-curing polyvinyl-siloxane for a patient infected with HIV. Describe the handling of the impression prior to the commencement of crown fabrication.

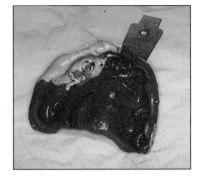

Figure 106

116 (a) Name the procedure shown in *Figure 107*.
(b) Discuss the indications and contraindications for the use of the technique.

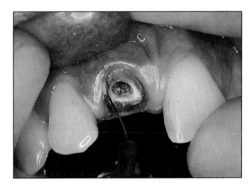

Figure 107

117 Two upper central incisors (*Figure 108*) were restored with jacket crowns 2 years previously. The patient now complains that the gums are sore and bleed readily.
(a) What is your diagnosis of the complaint and to what can the cause be attributed?
(b) How can the condition be resolved and how would you plan the necessary treatment?

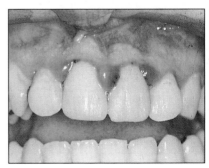

Figure 108

118 (a) What is 'cracked tooth syndrome'?
(b) How may the offending tooth be identified?

119 During the restoration of an MOD cavity in an elderly patient, the glass-ionomer (polyalkenoate) was deliberately externalised (arrowed) as shown in *Figure 109*,

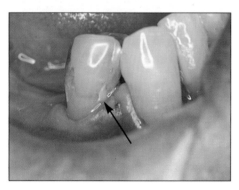

resulting in an 'open sandwich' restoration.
(a) Describe the rationale for this procedure.
(b) Are there any potential problems associated with the technique?
(c) Why was it justified in this patient?
(d) Which type of glass-ionomer would you use?

Figure 109

120 *Figure 110* is the fitting surface of a minimal-preparation bridge retainer.
(a) What type of retention has been produced on the fit surface?

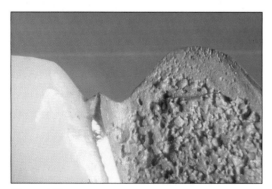

(b) How has it been created?
(c) Outline the advantages and disadvantages of this method of retention.
(d) Describe other methods by which retention can be provided.

Figure 110

121 The upper central incisors have been restored with porcelain veneers (*Figure 111*) without any tooth preparation having been carried out.

(a) What are the advantages and disadvantages of preparing teeth before porcelain veneer placement?

(b) What features require assessment during veneer try-in?

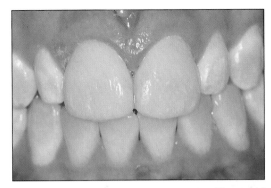

Figure 111

(c) Outline the essential stages to achieve satisfactory veneer cementation.

122 A 54-year-old patient attends your surgery with a mixture of worn buccal tooth surfaces and superimposed carious lesions (*Figure 112*). He is concerned about the appearance of his teeth.

(a) What are the possible aetiological factors that may have contributed to the condition?

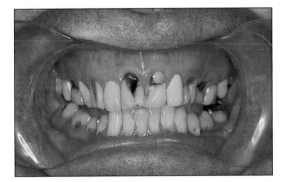

Figure 112

(b) How would you formulate a treatment plan for this patient?

(c) Describe possible treatment options that should be considered to achieve dental fitness.

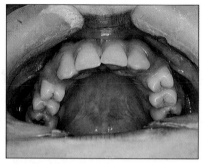

Figure 113

123 An 18-year-old girl has congenitally missing upper lateral incisors and the canines have been moved mesially (*Figure 113*) to fill the lateral spaces using an orthodontic appliance.
(a) What would be the treatment of choice to restore the residual spaces?
(b) Is the orthodontic movement of canines desirable in this type of case?
(c) At what stage would restorative treatment be appropriate?

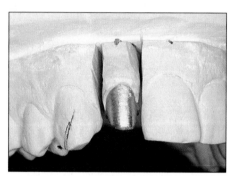

Figure 114

124 A metal–ceramic crown is to be made for the upper lateral incisor (*Figure 114*).
(a) Describe the different types of alloy that can be used for the metal substructure.
(b) Outline the laboratory stages in the construction of such a crown.
(c) How will the porcelain be retained to the metal?

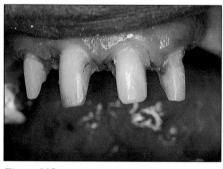

Figure 115

125 *Figure 115* shows four teeth that have been prepared for metal–ceramic crowns. The upper right lateral tooth has a composite core retained by a stainless steel parallel post.
(a) What are the advantages and disadvantages of this type of post and core?
(b) List the good and bad features of the other three preparations.

126 What criteria should you use in deciding whether to provide a restoration when early approximal caries shows in a premolar tooth on a bitewing radiograph?

127 An upper right canine (*Figure 116*) had a porcelain jacket crown fitted 6 years ago.
(a) Describe the condition associated with the lower teeth.
(b) What is the likely cause and how can it be avoided?

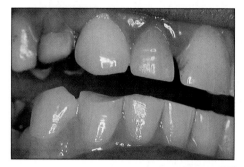

Figure 116

128 A patient complains of the repeated loss of a post crown (*Figure 117*) that replaces an upper lateral incisor tooth.
(a) Why does the restoration keep falling out?
(b) What factors may have contributed to the failure?
(c) How might the situation have been prevented?

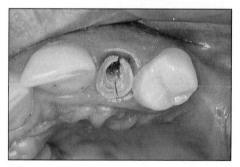

Figure 117

129 *Figure 118* shows the labial surfaces of a canine and premolar of a 53-year-old patient.
(a) Describe the appearance of the cervical aspect of the upper premolar. What is the lesion?
(b) How would you decide whether the lesion is active or arrested?
(c) Under what circumstances would you decide to place a filling?

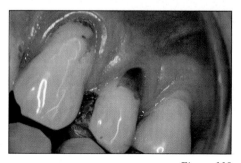

Figure 118

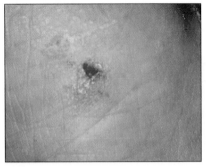

Figure 119

130 During routine operative treatment of a new patient you knock your hand against the bracket table, resulting in a deep penetrating injury (*Figure 119*) from a contaminated bur. Briefly describe the action you would take.

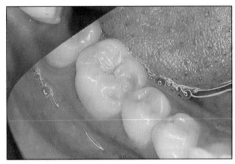

Figure 120

131 An 18-year-old patient complains of sensitivity from a tooth (*Figure 120*) when eating and drinking cold drinks.
(a) Describe the steps you would take to determine the cause of the tooth-substance loss.
(b) How would you manage the treatment of the tooth?

132 (a) When planning restorative dental care, what use can be made of non-vital teeth in the treatment plan?
(b) Outline the aspects that should be considered before determining the use of such teeth.
(c) Other than a history and clinical examination, indicate what information will be of use to you.

133 (a) Describe the features shown on the palatal aspect of the two crowns illustrated in *Figure 121*.
(b) Why have they been used?

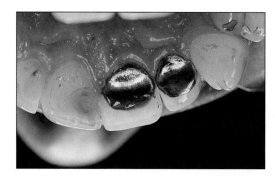

Figure 121

134 Resin-bonded ceramic crowns (*Figure 122*) were fitted 6 weeks ago. A ferric sulphate solution was used as part of a tissue-management regime when taking the working impression and later at the time of resin bonding.
(a) Why has the discoloration occurred at the margin?
(b) What is its significance?
(c) How can the occurrence be prevented?

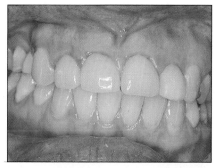

Figure 122

135 The upper right first premolar (*Figure 123*) has been restored with an MOD ceramic inlay which covers the weakened buccal cusp.
(a) Give the indications and contraindications for the use of tooth-coloured inlay/onlay restorations.
(b) What are the essential features of the preparations?
(c) Suggest alternative materials that could be employed to restore this tooth, indicating the important differences in cavity preparation that would be required.

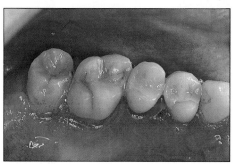

Figure 123

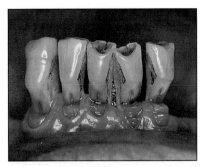

Figure 124

136 Your glass-ionomer (poly-alkenoate) restorations repeatedly fail on a patient (*Figure 124*).
(a) Suggest possible reasons for this failure.
(b) Describe means by which the problem could be overcome.
(c) What are the advantages of using glass-ionomer cement clinically?
(d) How does the material adhere to dentine?

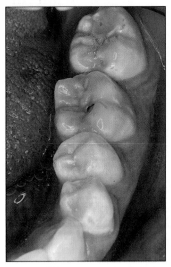

Figure 125

137 On a routine 6-month examination of a 20-year-old patient, occlusal caries was detected in an isolated fissure in the lower left first molar (*Figure 125*). No other restoration or caries was present in the mouth. The left bitewing radiograph is shown in *Figure 126*.
(a) What factors have contributed to this situation?
(b) How would you manage the lesion?
(c) What advice would you give to the patient?

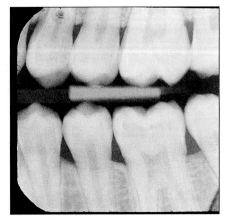

Figure 126

138 (a) Give the clinical indications for the placement of composite resin restorations in posterior teeth.
(b) What aspects of technique will ensure the success of such restorations?

139 The model shown in *Figure 127* has been made from two dissimilar materials.
(a) What is the technique called and from what materials has the model been constructed?
(b) How will it aid the production of the crowns?

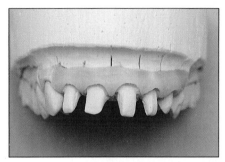

Figure 127

140 (a) Is a Black's Class II cavity described as one which:
(i)   Involves the occlusal surface and extends to the proximal surface.
(ii) Is in the proximal surface of molars and premolars.
(iii) Has caries involving the occlusal surface plus the mesial and/or distal surface.
(iv) Extends from the occlusal surface to the interproximal surface of a posterior tooth.
(b) In a Class II restoration which of the following factors are of importance to the health of the periodontal tissues?
(i)   Contour of the occlusal surface.
(ii) Design of the contact.
(iii) Contour and position of the cervical margin relative to the gingival tissue.
(iv) Surface smoothness of the restoration.
(v)   Marginal adaption of the restoration.
(c) At which stage in the preparation of a Class II cavity should carious dentine be removed from the pulpal floor?
(i)   As the first stage.
(ii) At any stage.
(iii) When the preparation is otherwise complete.

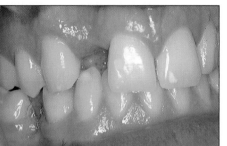

Figure 128

141 A young adult male patient seeks advice regarding the replacement of a missing upper right lateral incisor (*Figure 128*).
(a) What are the design options for the replacement of such a tooth by means of a bridge?
(b) What would influence your final choice of design?

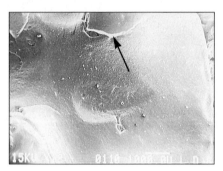

Figure 129

142 A scanning electron micrograph (*Figure 129*) shows two types of wear on the surface of a posterior composite. In the centre is an obvious scar, while at the edge of the restoration the enamel margin has been exposed (arrowed).
(a) What causes these types of wear?
(b) Give the terminology used to describe them in dentistry.
(c) Are these terms synonymous when used to describe the wear of teeth?

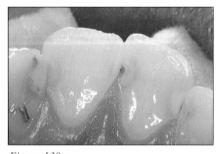

Figure 130

143 The palatal surfaces of the upper incisors of a 20-year-old are shown in *Figure 130*.
(a) What fillings are required in the upper left central incisor? From which aspect of the tooth would you gain access to the carious lesions?
(b) Why would it not be possible to manage these lesions by purely preventive procedures?
(c) Comment on the tooth-coloured filling on the mesial aspect of the upper lateral incisor. Would you replace the filling?
(d) What special test would you carry out before giving a local anaesthetic?
(e) Would you use a topical anaesthetic before giving a local anaesthetic?

144 Describe the possible adverse reactions which may arise following the application of the type of material shown in *Figure 131* to a traumatically exposed pulp in a mature permanent tooth.

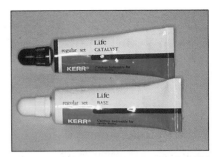

Figure 131

145 An endodontically treated tooth (*Figure 132*) now requires a core restoration. Discuss the advantages and disadvantages of the alternative forms of retention that are available.

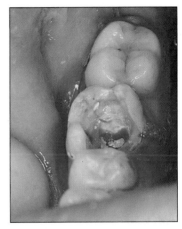

Figure 132

146 On routine clinical examination a symptom-free discoloured upper premolar is noticed (*Figure 133*).
(a) What investigations and tests are indicated?
(b) What is your differential diagnosis of the condition?
(c) Outline the treatment options?

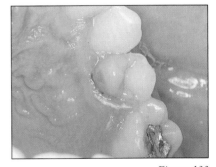

Figure 133

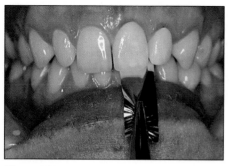

Figure 134

147 The upper left central and lateral incisor crowns (*Figure 134*) are being assessed prior to permanent cementation.
(a) What technique is being used?
(b) What other features should be checked at this appointment?

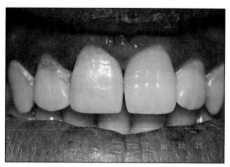

Figure 135

148 The incisal third of the distal corner of the upper right central incisor (*Figure 135*) has been restored.
(a) What material is most likely to have been used?
(b) What steps have been taken to match the aesthetics of the neighbouring tooth?
(c) Outline the stages of the placement technique, indicating the reasons for their inclusion.

149 You are using a hand-mixed anhydrous glass-ionomer (polyalkenoate) cement. Your assistant adds too much water to the mix to make the material more fluid.
(a) What are the components of an anhydrous glass-ionomer material?
(b) What effects will this alteration in powder:liquid (P:L) ratio have upon the setting characteristics and physical properties of the cement mass?
(c) What are the benefits of using encapsulated material?

150 Six months after placement of a direct cantilever bridge (*Figure 136*), replacing the upper first premolar using the upper second premolar and upper first molar as abutments, a patient complained of tenderness and bleeding from the gingivae in the area.
(a) What has contributed to the problem?
(b) How should this situation have been avoided?

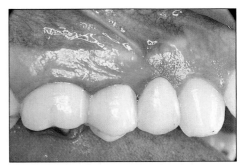

Figure 136

151 A healthy adult patient complains of pain in the upper left quadrant in which several large amalgam restorations have recently been placed. Describe the investigation, diagnosis and treatment of the patient.

152 (a) Describe the features of the occlusopalatal cavity in this upper first permanent molar (*Figure 137*).
(b) How and why should the cavity be modified?

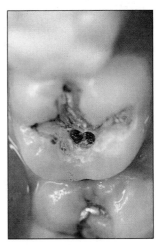

Figure 137

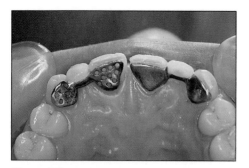

Figure 138

153 A patient has two minimum preparation (resin-retained) bridges (*Figure 138*).
(a) Describe the design of the one on the right and the mechanism for its retention.
(b) What are the alternative techniques by which the one on the left may be retained?
(c) Outline the advantages and disadvantages of the two different techniques employed to retain these bridges.

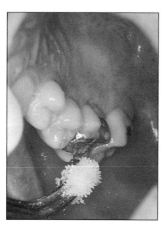

Figure 139

154 (a) What is the likely substance being applied to the heavily restored upper permanent molar on the pledget of cotton wool (*Figure 139*)?
(b) If no response is elicited, what are the possible explanations?

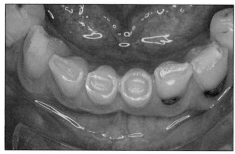

Figure 140

155 A patient has cupping of the dentine (*Figure 140*) associated with the lower incisors.
(a) Which term would you use to describe the condition and why?
(b) What material would you use to restore the defects?
(c) Describe any possible long-term iatrogenic effects of your treatment.

156 (a) What is the blue ring (*Figure 141*) between the premolar and molar?
(b) Why has it been placed?

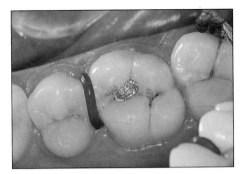

Figure 141

157 (a) What types of material used in operative dentistry are represented by the four products shown in *Figure 142*?
(b) Which is the most suitable as a routine pulp-capping material and why?
(c) What is the likely outcome if the other materials are used in this situation?

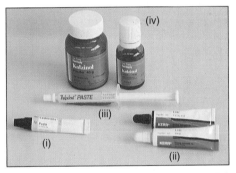

Figure 142

158 A patient is displeased with the appearance of a metal–ceramic crown (*Figure 143*) on the upper right central incisor.
(a) In remaking the restoration, what clinical and laboratory procedures may help to provide a more satisfactory restoration?
(b) What are the indications for the construction of a metal–ceramic crown?
(c) Describe alternative techniques for crown construction that should be considered before replacing the crown.

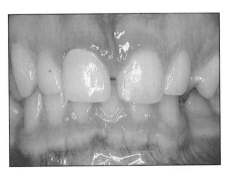

Figure 143

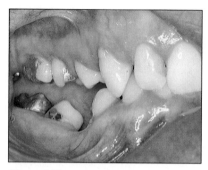

Figure 144

159 A 40-year-old female patient is concerned about the long-standing bilateral spaces between her posterior teeth when she bites. The occlusion on the right side is shown in *Figure 144* and the left is similar.
(a) What are the possible causes for the condition?
(b) Outline the investigations that are indicated to enable you to determine a suitable course of treatment.
(c) If the condition is determined to be iatrogenic, how should it have been prevented?

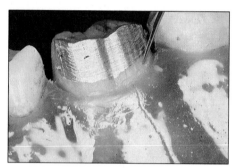

Figure 145

160 (a) Name the feature (*Figure 145*) of this full-crown preparation which is being examined with the aid of a probe.
(b) Why is it important?

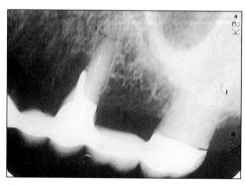

Figure 146

161 The toothache suffered by a patient (*Figure 146*) in the upper left posterior quadrant was typical of pulpitis.
(a) What is the likely cause of the pain?
(b) How may this be confirmed?
(c) What treatment possibilities should be considered?

162 A failed crown is shown in *Figure 147* and the corresponding tooth preparation in *Figure 148*.
(a) What material has been used to construct the core?
(b) Why has it failed?
(c) Under what conditions could this material be used safely?
(d) How would you prevent this problem from recurring when remaking the crown?

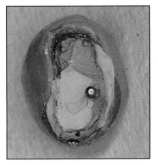

Figure 147

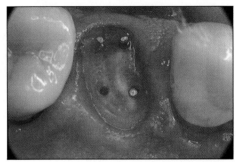

Figure 148

163 (a) Comment on the radiographic appearance (*Figure 149*) of the mesial surface of the lateral incisor.
(b) Which clinical procedure could have led to this appearance?
(c) How should this procedure be undertaken to overcome the problem?

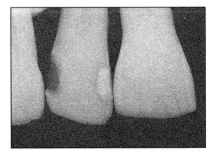

Figure 149

164 (a) What are the indications for the placement of porcelain veneers?
(b) In what situations are they contraindicated?
(c) How is the fitting surface of the veneer treated in order to facilitate bonding?

165 The buccal cusp of the upper second premolar has fractured (*Figure 150*) following the placement of a posterior composite resin restoration.

(a) Why may this have occurred?

(b) What steps could have been taken to minimise the risk of such an occurrence for a patient desiring a tooth-coloured posterior restoration?

(c) How would you now propose proceeding?

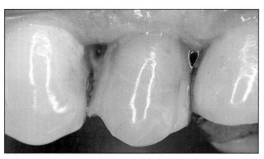

Figure 150

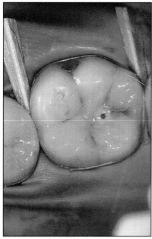

Figure 151

166 A first molar tooth (*Figure 151*) in a patient aged 22 has been isolated with rubber dam and dried. The caries in the distal fossa is obvious.

(a) How confident would you be of diagnosing this caries in the dental chair without isolation and drying?

(b) How confident would you be of diagnosing this caries if you were examining the patient in their own home with portable equipment?

(c) How extensive do you anticipate the caries will be in dentine?

(d) Why do you think the enamel has not given way, exposing a larger cavity?

167 (a) Describe the structures that the needle passes through when administering an inferior dental block to enable operative dentistry to be undertaken on the lower left first molar.

(b) Which other cranial nerve may be inadvertently anaesthetised at the same time?

(c) Outline the clinical procedures you would adopt should signs and/or symptoms indicate that this has occurred.

168 Which of the following statements are correct?
(a) When placing a Class II amalgam restoration wedging of the matrix band:
    (i)   Is always necessary.
    (ii) Assists in achieving the correct contour for the proximal surface of the restoration.
    (iii) Enables an adequate condensation load to be applied to the amalgam.
    (iv) Prevents a gingival overhang.
    (v) Compensates for the thickness of the matrix band.
(b) Amalgam restorations exhibit 'ditched margins' because:
    (i)   There is inadequate extension for prevention.
    (ii) The isthmus is too narrow.
    (iii) Amelo-dentinal junction caries has not been removed.
    (iv) Cavity margins have not been finished.
    (v) There is an excessively thick cement base.
    (vi) The carving is faulty.
    (vii) Of moisture contamination.
(c) When polishing an amalgam restoration the objectives are to:
    (i)   Remove slight marginal excess.
    (ii) Reduce the likelihood of surface stagnation.
    (iii) Improve its appearance.
    (iv) Carve the surface anatomy.
    (v) Eliminate the consequences of previous faulty manipulation.

169 (a) Describe the appearance of the two upper central incisors, shown in *Figure 152*, which have sustained trauma.
(b) Suggest possible reasons for their appearance.
(c) What are the potential long-term complications of this form of care?

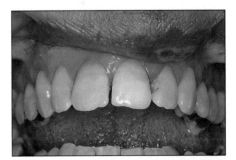

Figure 152

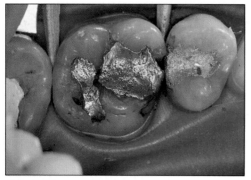

Figure 153

170 *Figure 153* shows an upper premolar and molar in a 22-year-old patient.
(a) Would you replace the mesio-occlusal restoration in the upper first molar?
(b) Why is there a shiny spot on the amalgam restoration in the premolar?
(c) Why has a wedge been placed on the mesial aspect of the upper first molar?

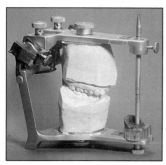

Figure 154

171 The plaster of Paris used for the articulation of the study casts shown in *Figure 154* was mixed with an aqueous solution containing potassium sulphate, borax and alizarin red.
(a) What is the common name for such a solution?
(b) Describe the properties these additives give the plaster which are of advantage in the articulation of study casts.

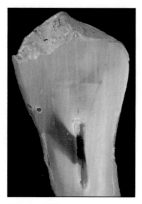

Figure 155

172 An extracted tooth (*Figure 155*) has been restored using a posterior composite and a dentine bonding system.
(a) Name the phenomenon that is shown.
(b) What is its clinical significance and how may it be minimised?
(c) Give other methods by which the phenomenon can be demonstrated.

173 A 45-year-old male patient requests that his upper front two teeth (*Figure 156*) be restored.
(a) What is your diagnosis of the condition?
(b) How should treatment proceed? Indicate any difficulties that you can foresee in the restoration of these teeth.

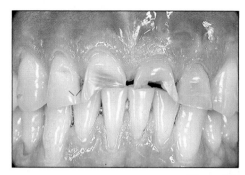

Figure 156

174 (a) What is the cause of this soft-tissue lesion (*Figure 157*) in the edentulous area?
(b) How may it be prevented from recurring?

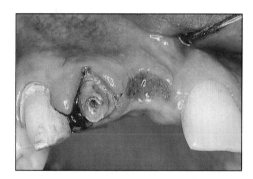

Figure 157

175 A scanning electron micrograph (*Figure 158*) depicts considerable wear associated with the palatal extension of a posterior composite.
(a) Which process has caused wear at this site?
(b) Why is it accentuated in buccal and lingual extensions?
(c) How can contouring of the restoration affect the process?
(d) How would you manage the case?

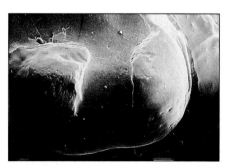

Figure 158

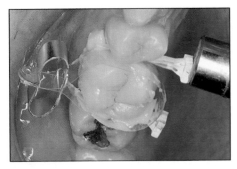

Figure 159

176 A stage in the fitting of a resin-bonded ceramic inlay is shown in *Figure 159*.
(a) Describe what is shown in the picture.
(b) Why is the procedure necessary?
(c) What short- and long-term problems may result if this procedure is not carried out as shown?

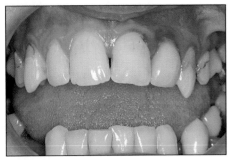

Figure 160

177 A patient attends your surgery complaining of gingival tenderness and bleeding associated with a recently cemented crown on the upper left lateral incisor (*Figure 160*).
(a) What are the possible aetiological factors for the problem?
(b) What investigations would you undertake?
(c) How would you manage the patient's discomfort?

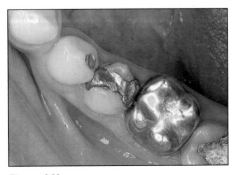

Figure 161

178 At a routine dental examination, a lower left second premolar (*Figure 161*) was charted as a failed amalgam restoration.
(a) What criteria would you apply in diagnosing a failed amalgam restoration?
(b) Describe, giving reasons, how you would treat such a case.

179 (a) What are the indications and contraindications that should be considered before recommending a bridge to a patient?
(b) Indicate the information that you would require before advising a patient how best to replace a missing tooth.

180 Six months after the placement of two adjacent Class II posterior composites (*Figure 162*) a patient complains of occasional soreness in the area.
(a) What is the most likely reason for the complaint?
(b) Describe any other signs that may be present.
(c) How may the problem be avoided?
(d) Discuss how you would manage the case.
(e) What is the cause of the small round defect (arrowed)?

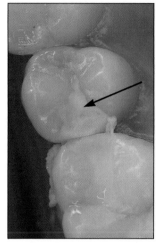

Figure 162

181 *Figure 163* demonstrates posterior full veneer crowns constructed in gold and as metal–ceramic restorations.
(a) Give the factors that are likely to influence the choice between these two forms of restoration.
(b) In what ways will the preparation for a metal–ceramic crown differ from the full gold crown preparation?
(c) Describe, with their advantages and disadvantages, the various finishing lines that can be employed for metal–ceramic preparation margins.

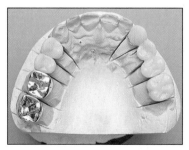

Figure 163

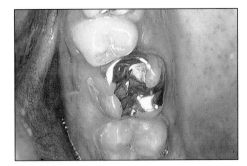

Figure 164

182 Set amalgam restorations should be finished (*Figure 164*).
(a) How and when should this be undertaken?
(b) What benefits does the procedure confer?

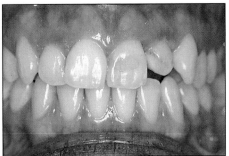

Figure 165

183 Both the upper left central and lateral incisors (*Figure 165*) are vital and exhibit no radiographic abnormality. Suggest a suitable treatment plan to improve the appearance of these teeth.

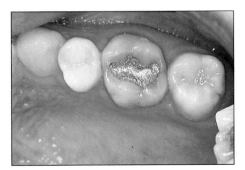

Figure 166

184 (a) What are the possible causes for the severe discoloration of the tooth tissue of the upper molar shown in *Figure 166*?
(b) Would you replace the filling?

185 (a) What is the device (*Figure 167*) that has been added to the lower member of this semi-adjustable articulator?
(b) Describe its purpose.

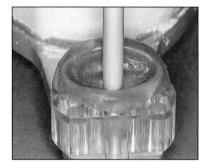

Figure 167

186 A patient (*Figure 168*) has recently had to have the anterior portion of a fixed–fixed bridge, retained by the upper canines and first premolars, sectioned and removed. The upper left first premolar retainer has also been removed.
(a) Name the condition that can be seen and describe why it may have occurred.
(b) How would you proceed clinically?

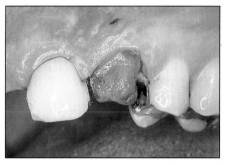

Figure 168

187 During your first exam-ination of a young adult patient, discoloration of the fissures of two molar teeth (*Figure 169*) is noticed. There has been no other caries experience.
(a) How can you determine if any treatment is indicated?
(b) What treatment options are available to you?

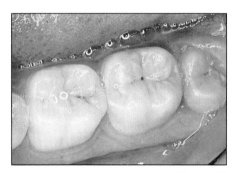

Figure 169

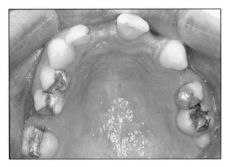

Figure 170

188 A patient (*Figure 170*) requests the provision of a fixed restoration to replace his removable partial denture.
(a) Outline the factors that should be taken into account before advising the patient.
(b) What preliminary investigations would you undertake?
(c) Indicate, with reasons, which would be the preferred abutment teeth and design of fixed bridgework.

189 (a) Describe the distinguishing aspects of toothache caused by a hyperaemic pulp.
(b) How may the offending tooth be identified and the diagnosis confirmed?

190 Upper incisor teeth (*Figure 171*) have been prepared to receive a resin-bonded bridge.
(a) Under the circumstances what is unusual about the anterior occlusion?

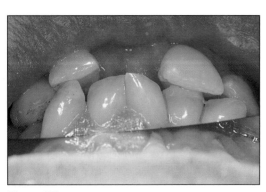

(b) What treatment has been undertaken on the occluding lower teeth and why?
(c) Describe how this will have been undertaken.
(d) Indicate any difficulties that might be experienced if this stage is omitted.

Figure 171

191 This glass-ionomer (polyalkenoate) cement restoration (*Figure 172*) contains metal particles within the glass of the cement.
(a) Describe the function of the metal particles.
(b) Which metals have been used in this role?
(c) Discuss the indications for the clinical use of these materials.

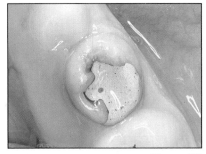

Figure 172

192 You are attempting to fit a metal–ceramic crown (*Figure 173*) but find it will not seat. What checks would you make (and in what order) to ascertain the cause of the problem?

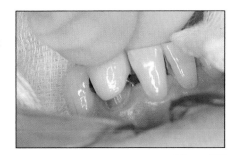

Figure 173

193 A 14-year-old patient attends your surgery with heavily discoloured and worn teeth (*Figure 174*). Several cusps have been lost and have been temporarily restored with glass-ionomer (polyalkenoate) cement.
(a) What specific questions would you ask in the history?
(b) What is the differential diagnosis?
(c) Describe the treatment alternatives.

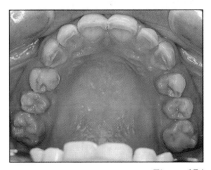

Figure 174

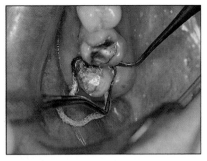

Figure 175

194 *Figure 175* shows gingival retraction cord being placed around a full-veneer crown preparation on the upper right second molar.
(a) Outline the indications for this procedure.
(b) What types of cord/medicaments are available for this purpose?

195 (a) How does the shape of amalgam alloy particles affect the properties of set amalgam?
(b) What effect does increasing the copper content of the alloy have on the set amalgam?
(c) Describe the overall changes of dimension which occur when a modern amalgam alloy is mixed with mercury and allowed to set.

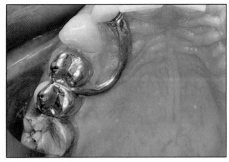

Figure 176

196 (a) What is the type of restoration that is shown in *Figure 176*?
(b) Are there any features of the design that make it inappropriate?
(c) Given the information that, other than the missing lateral incisor, the upper arch is intact suggest an alternative means for replacing the lost tooth.

197 The restoration in the lower first molar shown in *Figure 177* is a hybrid posterior composite, while that in the second molar is a glass-ionomer (polyalkenoate).
(a) Describe what is wrong with both restorations.
(b) What was the primary problem in this case?
(c) How would you manage the situation?

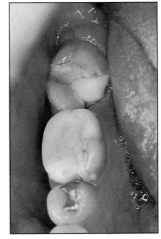

Figure 177

198 The occlusal surface of this completed full-veneer crown (*Figure 178*) has been treated prior to its transportation to the clinic for try-in.
(a) What treatment has it received?
(b) What is its purpose?

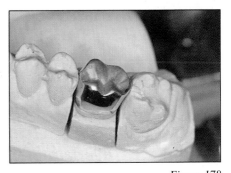

Figure 178

199 Describe the advantages and disadvantages of using the impression material shown in *Figure 179* for crown and bridgework.

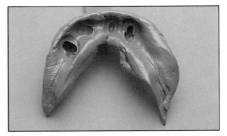

Figure 179

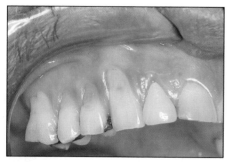

Figure 180

200 (a) What is the condition that can be seen associated with the upper right canine and premolars shown in *Figure 180*?
(b) If it is decided that restoration is appropriate, suggest the most suitable method.
(c) Indicate the advantages of the material(s) that you would consider using.

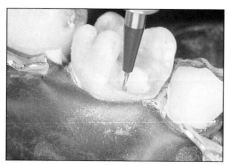

Figure 181

201 (a) Describe the clinical procedure that is being demonstrated in *Figure 181*.
(b) What are the principles involved in its use?

202 (a) What factors need to be favourable before considering pulp capping?
(b) Outline the clinical sequence that you would adopt when undertaking this procedure.
(c) What would lead you to suspect that the treatment had not been successful?

203 A patient complains of severe sensitivity from his lower incisor teeth (*Figure 182*). He wears an upper complete denture with ceramic anterior teeth and is complaining of pain and clicking from his temporomandibular joints. The lower teeth are severely worn and several attempts have been made to control the sensitivity without success.

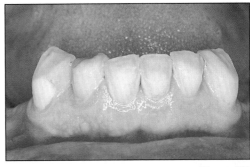

Figure 182

(a) Why are the anterior teeth so worn?
(b) What treatment options would you consider to help the patient?
(c) How could a dental laboratory help in planning the future treatment?

204 The cervical restoration in the upper left lateral incisor shown in *Figure 183* has failed.
(a) Describe the possible ways in which the tooth may be restored both aesthetically and conservatively.
(b) What are the advantages and disadvantages associated with each approach considered?

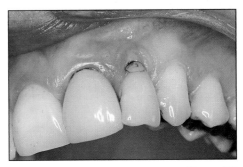

Figure 183

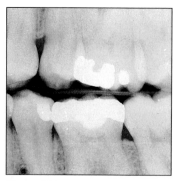

Figure 184

205 (a) Describe the restoration that is present in the lower left second premolar shown in *Figure 184*.
(b) What clinical technique has been used?
(c) What are the indications and advantages of this form of restoration?
(d) Which material could you employ in the technique?
(e) What technical problems might you encounter?

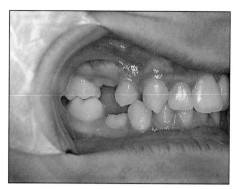

Figure 185

206 A young adult patient is concerned about the situation that can be seen developing in the lower right quadrant (*Figure 185*).
(a) What are the reasons for the condition having developed?
(b) Suggest, with reasons, ways by which it would be possible to establish full occlusion.

207 An extracted tooth (*Figure 186*) has a very deep labial notch and a shallower lingual depression, mostly in dentine.
(a) What is said to be the most common aetiology of this type of labial notch?
(b) Could the same aetiology explain the lingual depression?

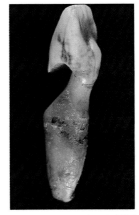

Figure 186

208 (a) Which of the current elastomeric impression materials shows the best dimensional stability?
(b) Are there any factors associated with the setting times of the elastomers which can have an adverse effect on their performance?
(c) Which of the elastomeric impression materials exhibits the greatest tear resistance?

209 A patient, who has recently given up smoking, is concerned about staining of the lower incisor teeth (*Figure 187*).
(a) Give the term used to describe the condition and state how it varies from the lesion shown in *Figure 140*.
(b) How would you manage the situation?
(c) The lesions shown in these figures are becoming more common—why?

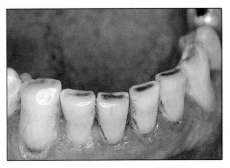

Figure 187

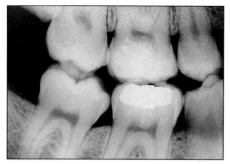

Figure 188

210 (a) Comment on the radiographic appearances of the restorations in the first molar teeth (*Figure 188*).
(b) Why should posterior filling materials be radiopaque?

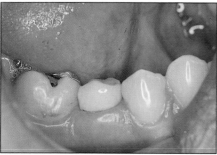

Figure 189

211 A patient complains that the crown on a lower premolar (*Figure 189*) keeps falling off.
(a) What is the main reason for this?
(b) What are likely to be contributory causes?
(c) How could the problem be overcome if the tooth was:
    (i) Non-vital?
    (ii) Vital?

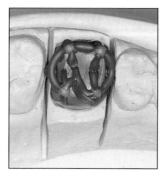

Figure 190

212 (a) What is the technical procedure (*Figure 190*) in progress on the occlusal surface of this full-veneer crown die?
(b) Outline the stages of the technique.
(c) What are the advantages conferred by this approach?

213 A patient attends your surgery complaining about the discoloration of their teeth (*Figure 191*), which have been treated unsuccessfully by enamel microabrasion.
(a) What agents are necessary to carry out the procedure?
(b) Which conditions are most amenable to treatment by this technique?
(c) Why has it been unsuccessful in this case?

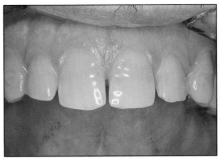

Figure 191

214 Outline the general and dental problems that may be encountered when providing restorative care for elderly patients with a surviving natural dentition.

215 (a) Name the condition that can be seen on the labial surface of the two upper central incisors shown in *Figure 192*.
(b) What is the likely aetiology?
(c) How would you propose managing the case?

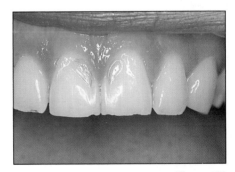

Figure 192

216 When examining a patient what information or observation might lead you to suspect that a tooth was non-vital?

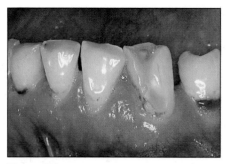

Figure 193

217 A porcelain veneer has been lost from the buccal surface of a lower left canine (*Figure 193*). There is some residual bonding resin left on the surface of the tooth with failure at the resin–veneer interface.
(a) What may have been responsible for the failure?
(b) How should the fit surface of porcelain veneers be treated to ensure a durable bond between the veneer and the resin?

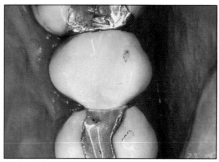

Figure 194

218 *Figure 194* shows a mesio-occlusal-distal composite resin restoration on an upper premolar.
(a) What problems are associated with the placement of this type of material?
(b) Describe service problems which may become apparent following its use.
(c) Upon what criteria would you base a decision to use this material?

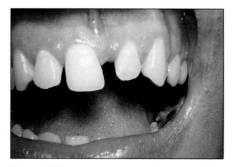

Figure 195

219 (a) Describe the condition shown in *Figure 195*.
(b) How might the case be managed and discuss the problems involved.

220 A 22-year-old patient has extensive tooth wear (*Figure 196*) that is clearly not the result of abrasion (physical wear from an external agent such as a toothbrush) but is likely to have resulted from a combination of erosion (chemical dissolution of the surface of the tooth) and attrition (physical wear from the opposing teeth).

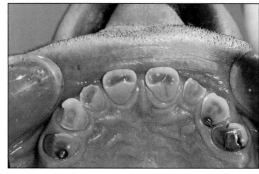

Figure 196

(a) How do you establish the differential diagnosis?
(b) What are the treatment options?
(c) List your criteria for choosing between them.

221 (a) The articulator illustrated in *Figure 197* is of what category?
(b) What adjustable elements does it incorporate?
(c) Describe the clinical records that are required to mount the casts and set the articulator controls.

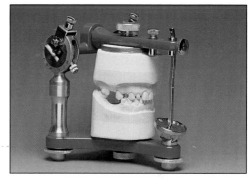

Figure 197

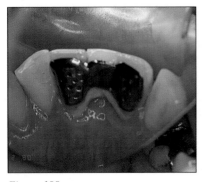

Figure 198

222 The bridge shown in *Figure 198*, which was made to replace a small denture several years ago, has delighted the patient.
(a) Name the type of bridge that has been used.
(b) Describe the deficiencies that can be seen and state how they could have been avoided.
(c) What sort of material is used to cement these bridges?
(d) Give the advantages of this design of bridge over those more recently developed.

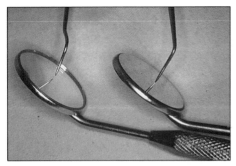

Figure 199

223 (a) What is the difference between the reflecting surfaces of the two mirrors shown in *Figure 199*?
(b) What advantage may the mirror on the right confer?

224 A bitewing radiograph (*Figure 200*) shows gross caries in the upper left first molar in a 19-year-old patient who was born and brought up in an area which has fluoridated water. Only limited signs of caries could be observed clinically.
(a) Account for the lack of clinical signs.
(b) Describe your management of the gross caries.

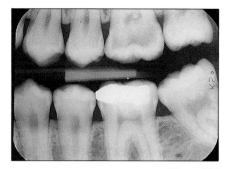

Figure 200

225 A large pin-retained restoration (*Figure 201*) was placed 12 months ago to replace a fractured buccal cusp in an upper first premolar. With a metal–matrix band in place, the composite was packed and cured in increments from the occlusal surface.
(a) What is the cause of the brown bands on the buccal surface?

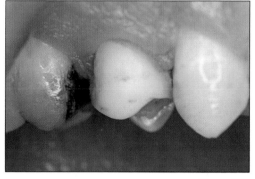

Figure 201

(b) How could the problem have been avoided?
(c) What other features are recognisable in the illustration?
(d) What is the cause of this problem?
(e) Do you consider that this restoration is a legitimate use for posterior composite. If so—why?

ANSWERS

1 (a) By definition the term 'high copper' implies over 6% Cu (by weight) in the alloy powder. However, in individual materials there may be up to 30% Cu.
(b) There should be less corrosion because there is less γ_2 in the set material.
(c) During setting all amalgams nucleate $Ag_2Hg_3(\gamma_1)$. Low-copper amalgams also nucleate $Sn_{7-8}Hg(\gamma_2)$. However, the high-copper materials nucleate Cu_6Sn_5 (η') in preference to γ_2. The η' phase is less susceptible to corrosion than γ_2.
(d) No. Research has indicated that some high-copper amalgams still form some γ_2 as well as γ_1 and η'.
(e)
- *Dispersed alloys* where the copper is present as separate Ag_3Cu particles in the powder. These are sometimes referred to as high-copper admixed (HCA) alloys.
- *Ternary alloys* where the silver, tin and copper have been formed into a single ternary alloy. These are sometimes referred to as high-copper single composition (HCSC) alloys.

2 (a) The teeth appear healthy. There is an obvious stained fissure in the lower first molar but no evidence of a cavity.
(b) When the teeth are examined they should be clean, dry and well lit so that subtle changes in the appearance of the tooth tissue can be appreciated by the operator. Magnification can help the dentist see clearly and becomes more important as middle age is approached. A sharp probe may be helpful to remove plaque from fissures gently but should not be jabbed into the fissure system as this may cause a break in an otherwise intact enamel surface.
(c) Fibre-optic transillumination and a bitewing radiograph may both aid diagnosis.
(d) Rubber dam has been placed because the radiograph (see *Figure 15*) shows a large lesion in dentine in the lower first molar which is now to be restored.

3 (a) Transillumination.
(b) Transillumination may have a useful diagnostic application for:
- *The detection of incomplete tooth fractures* (as in the case illustrated). Incomplete coronal fractures are often difficult to visualise under normal clinical lighting conditions. The application of a strong localised light source may allow easy visualisation of a fracture as a dark line, or as a line of transition where the light is prevented by the fracture from passing further into the crown of the tooth.
- *The diagnosis of caries.* Transillumination may enhance visualisation of stained, carious dentine, especially beneath seemingly intact pits and fissures, and in interproximal regions.
- *As a supplementary aid in pulp vitality testing.* Non-vital teeth which present no noticeable discoloration when viewed under normal clinical lighting conditions may show a marked difference in translucency when transilluminated. Visualisation of resorptive defects affecting the coronal tissue of teeth may also be enhanced.
- *The location of fine root canal orifices.* Transillumination may assist in the identification of fine root-canal entrances which are often difficult to locate with normal clinical lighting.

4 (a) The articulator pictured is a Denar Mk II (Plus) semi-adjustable arcon (*ar*ticulated *con*dyle) articulator. In this form of articulator the mandibular element has a representation of the condyles and these articulate with the 'glenoid fossa' elements of the maxillary component.

(b) The articulator can be used for:
- Diagnostic mounting of study casts to allow examination of occlusal contacts in the retruded contact position and analysis of tooth contacts during excursive movements of the mounted models.
- The articulator can also be used during the fabrication of cast and porcelain restorations, thus ensuring correct tooth contacts in occlusion and mandibular movements.

(c) Although this articulator allows adjustment for the condylar angle and immediate and progressive side-shift, a number of limitations exist. These include:
- A straight condylar path to the articulator, whereas in the patient this is a non-uniform sigmoid curve.
- The articulator intercondylar distance is fixed at an average value and no adjustment is possible to the rear or superior wall of the glenoid fossa element of the articulator.

5 (a) The appearance of the clean dentine around the small bleeding point suggests that there has been a traumatic exposure of the mesial buccal pulp horn during cavity preparation. The initial treatment should involve the isolation of the tooth, preferably by rubber dam, and, as the exposure is small in size, it should be directly pulp capped with a setting calcium hydroxide material. The patient should be informed of the occurrence.

(b) A lack of retention is likely to be the main problem in restoring this tooth. Besides the placement of a base, some form of additional retention will therefore be required. This can most satisfactorily be provided by the use of pins carefully sited to avoid further traumatic injury to the pulp or periodontium.

(c) The final restoration is likely to be a full veneer crown. It should be appreciated, however, that the crown height is already limited and further reduction to gain adequate occlusal clearance may jeopardise the retention of the final restoration. Careful assessment of the occlusion and the use of retention grooves should allow a satisfactory crown to be placed. A full crown is preferred to a three-quarter as full coverage will impart additional retention. In this position in the mouth a metal–ceramic crown is unlikely to be indicated, especially as additional tooth reduction would be required if this option was selected.

(d) Because of the pulp exposure, monitoring of the vitality of the tooth will be required at regular intervals. If, on one of these occasions, no response is obtained, a periapical radiograph will be necessary to confirm clinical findings. If apical pathology is present, a decision will be required whether to initiate endodontic therapy or extract the tooth.

6 (a) There are areas of radiolucency on the external root surface of the left central incisor with loss of the associated lamina dura. If the tooth is firm clinically then the loss of lamina dura may indicate ankylosis of the root dentine to the alveolar bone. The root canal appears intact. The condition is external resorption.

(b) The exact mechanism is poorly understood. The most likely aetiology is traumatic injury to the tooth but some cases have been reported as idiopathic, where no agent has been identified. External resorption may also be associated with obvious root fracture or with the reimplantation or transplantation of teeth. Where no obvious root fracture exists after trauma, it is possible that microcracks have been created in the root dentine which are sufficient to stimulate osteoclastic activity. In the fracture of a bone, the resorption of the bone ends is the usual preliminary to new matrix formation and calcific healing. If this analogy is accepted in the case of dentine, there is no mechanism for healing, except by a fibrous tissue zone, but the precursor reaction still occurs. In the case of resorption associated with reimplantation, the resorption is probably a foreign body response to root dentine which has lost its living cementum cells.

(c) In the short term, when the resorption has been identified, an attempt should be made to arrest it by carrying out root canal therapy and filling the canal with a non-setting calcium hydroxide (in propylene glycol). It is assumed that hydroxyl ions diffuse through the dentine to the root surface and create conditions of increased alkalinity which are unfavourable to continued osteoclast activity. This treatment may slow or arrest the resorption. When the tooth appears stable, the calcium hydroxide may be replaced with a conventional root filling.

In the long term the prognosis depends on how much root is lost. If the tooth remains firm with a reduced root length, this almost certainly indicates ankylosis. Provided the tooth is functional and of good appearance, this is not a problem. However, if a restoration is required difficulties may arise. There may, for example, be a reduced root canal to retain a post. The presence of the resorption may prevent proper restoration and then the best plan will be to extract the tooth (usually with difficulty if it is ankylosed) and provide a bridge or partial denture.

A further complication occurs if an area of resorption communicates with the gingival crevice. This seems to be prone to infection and pocket formation. The prognosis then is very poor.

7 (a) Physical trauma to the tooth.
(b) The blow probably severed pulpal vessels, causing a severe pulpal haemorrhage, and also the apical vein, thus preventing venous return. Breakdown products from the pulpal clot, similar to those in a bruise elsewhere in the body, would enter the dentinal tubules and be visible through the translucent enamel.

8 (a) The gel may contain either hydrofluoric acid or acidulated phosphate fluoride as the active ingredient. Both chemicals will etch ceramic surfaces by selectively removing certain phases, depending upon their distribution in the material. The etching process increases the surface area and produces microscopic undercuts into which resin penetrates, forming a strong mechanical bond. Etching times vary from 90 s to 4 min and rubber dam is mandatory when using buffered hydrofluoric acid. Prior to the use of ceramic etchants orthophosphoric acid, which simply cleaned the surface without etching, was recommended.
(b) Visible light cured or dual cured resins may be bonded to etched ceramic surfaces. The final restoration may be a direct composite resin where the lost fragment is small. If the fractured fragment is retained by the patient and fits the fractured surface well, it may be rebonded into place, thus restoring the original aesthetics. A third possibility is to fabricate a new ceramic facing, or veneer in a dental laboratory.
- Fractured ceramic surfaces may be rather smooth and benefit from grit blasting with 50 μm alumina to clean and roughen the surface prior to etching using an intra-oral grit blaster.
- Following etching, an organosilane compound should be applied to the surface to enhance the resin bond. Silanes will promote a strong resin bond without etching, but the durability of the bond is uncertain.
- The effectiveness of the silane coupling agent is improved if a drying agent (acetone or ethanol) is applied after air drying.
- An unfilled resin should be applied before any final restorative resin or luting agent to promote wetting of the etched ceramic surface.

9 (a) Photoinitiated composites are single component pastes and the polymerisation process is activated by an external energy source. The α-diketone initiator (generally camphor quinone) absorbs energy from a visible (470 nm—blue light) light source. The ketone absorbs energy and reacts with an amine (added to the system to enhance the effect of the light-sensitive catalyst) to produce free radicals.
(b) The 'wand' type handpiece has a fibre-optic flexible cable which can be damaged, leading to loss of efficiency. There is only one size of curing tip and this cannot be autoclaved. The gun unit has a single light-connecting rod which can be autoclaved and

exchanged for tips with different diameters. Gun units suffer from the disadvantages of weight, noise and heat.

10 (a) In the healthy unmedicated adult there are few effects on salivary flow. There is a small reduction in resting secretion by the sub-mandibular glands and some fall in stimulated flow rates in the minor glands. This is likely to be a result of elevated levels of cholinergic tone in older subjects, where an anti-cholinergic challenge has a more profound effect upon salivary flow than in a younger population.

(b) Salivary flow can be impaired by either destruction of glandular tissue or chemical interference in the secretory mechanism. Gland destruction is bought about either by autoimmune disease (Sjögren's syndrome), when it is associated with dry eyes and rheumatoid arthritis, or by accidental irradiation of salivary tissue during radiotherapy for head and neck cancer. Interference with secretion is brought about by a wide range of pharmacological agents which either have an anticholinergic effect (e.g. tricyclic antidepressants) or which interfere with water balance (e.g. diuretics).

Dry mouth will cause:
• Painful, sensitive mucosae.
• Difficulty in chewing/swallowing.
• A tendency for oral infections, often fungal in origin.
• A characteristic pattern of decay involving exposed dentine surfaces either at the cervical margin or even on incisal edges.
• Difficulty in tolerating dentures that are mucosally borne; denture retention will also be reduced.

(c) An artificial saliva can be used to replace or supplement saliva present in the mouth. It should be sufficiently viscous that it is retained for a reasonable length of time in the oral cavity for a given application. It should be bland in flavour and texture, and should *not* contain fermentable carbohydrate or acids as a gustatory stimulus to salivary secretion. It should have neutral pH, preferably be saturated for calcium and phosphate, and contain fluoride in an available form.

11 (a) The section has been stained with haematoxylin and eosin, which is a routine, general-purpose histological stain.

(b) There is an acute inflammatory reaction in the pulp tissue beneath the cavity.

(c) Some disturbance of the odontoblastic layer has occurred and the cell nuclei have passed into the tubules. This is indicative of some form of physical trauma to the tooth and dehydration.

(d) While the histological appearance does not always directly relate to the clinical symptoms, in this case the tooth was tender to percussion and the patient had been kept awake the previous night.

12 (a)
    (i)   Shoulder.
    (ii) Bevelled shoulder.
    (iii) Chamfer.
    (iv) Knife-edge.

(b)
• The *shoulder* preparation is the finishing line of choice for porcelain jacket crown preparations. The edge strength of porcelain is low; therefore, a butt joint is required. The shoulder provides resistance to occlusal forces and minimises stresses in the porcelain. The margin can be easily read on both impression and die. The main disadvantage is that any inaccuracies in the fit of the crown will be reproduced at the margin, resulting in an increased thickness of cement lute.

- The *bevelled shoulder* allows a sliding fit to occur at the margin and therefore may be used on the proximal box of inlays and the occlusal shoulder of mandibular $\frac{3}{4}$ crowns. It may also be used for the labial margins of metal–ceramic crowns. Providing these margins are placed just into the gingival crevice little display of metal will be noted. In posterior quadrants of the mouth, where aesthetics are less important, the length of the bevel may be increased.
- The *chamfer* preparation is the preferred finishing line for veneer gold restorations. The resultant casting has sufficient marginal strength; at the same time it allows the sliding joint at its periphery to minimise the gap between the tooth and preparation, thus reducing the thickness of the cement lute. A well-prepared chamfer margin combines the advantage of an easily definable margin, on both the impression and die, with minimal tooth preparation.
- The *knife-edge* preparation provides, theoretically, the best finishing margin for cast gold restorations, allowing burnishing and adaptation of the gold. In practice this finishing line is difficult to read on both the impression and die and may lead to inaccurate extension and also distortion of the wax pattern, and subsequent casting, as a result of the thin wax. It also offers least marginal strength to the casting.

13 (a) The restoration in the molar has failed because:
- The distal isthmus region exhibits bulk fracture.
- There are a number of cracks/fracture lines radiating from the mesial isthmus region.
- Discoloration of the occluso-buccal cavosurface margin and adjacent enamel suggests the presence of caries at this site.
- General gross loss of surface contour and bulk discoloration of the restoration indicates that it was probably inadequately polymerised when placed.

(b)
- Posterior composite resin restorations are frequently indicated in the treatment of occlusal carious lesions which allow conservative preparations (the preventive resin restoration).
- They may also be indicated for the restoration of Class II cavities in premolar teeth where the appearance is very important, the cavity margins are in enamel, and the occlusal contacts are on enamel.
- Posterior composites may also be considered for use as interim or 'holding' restorations for endodontically treated posterior teeth (cuspal fracture with MOD amalgams is very common).

14 (a) The functions of a base material are to:
- Provide protection for the dentine and pulp from chemical and physical trauma.
- Reduce a deep cavity to appropriate depth for filling.
- Support undermined enamel.
- Eliminate undercuts when necessary.
- Confer resistance form.
- Provide an intermediary layer suitable for bonding.

(b) Materials that can be employed include:
- Modified zinc oxide/eugenol cements.
- Ethoxybenzoic acid cements.
- Zinc phosphate cements.
- Zinc polycarboxylate cements.
- Glass-ionomer (polyalkenoate) cements.
- Calcium hydroxide.

(c) *Modified zinc oxide/eugenol* cements are satisfactory for basing large and complex cavities. They are able to withstand the pressures of amalgam condensation and, as they have minimal effects on the pulp, they can be applied directly to the floor of deep cavities without the need for sublining.

Ethoxybenzoic acid (EBA) cements are modified zinc oxide/eugenol cements with the addition of fused quartz or alumina and hydrogenated rosin. They have increased compressive and tensile strengths with physical properties similar to the phosphates but with less irritant effects on the pulp, which allows them to be placed in deep cavities without a sublining.

Zinc phosphate cements provide good pulpal protection from thermal, electrical and pressure stimuli but may damage the pulp as a result of an initial low pH. This, however, can be of benefit as it provides an antibacterial effect which reduces the numbers of viable microorganisms in the cavity floor and thus decreases pulpal irritation. The materials are susceptible to an alteration in water content—an increase accelerates the speed of reaction and reduces the physical properties. Maximum powder should be incorporated into the mix so that it gains maximum strength to resist the packing forces required during the placement of amalgam.

Zinc polycarboxylate cements have a compressive strength comparable to that of zinc phosphate while the tensile strength is higher; its final strength is dependent on the powder/liquid ratio, with more powder giving greater strength. These cements tend to absorb water, are slightly more soluble than zinc phosphate, and adhere to tooth substance unless the surface is contaminated with saliva. The strength of set material is sufficient for amalgam condensation and its effect on the pulp is mild enough to eliminate the need for a sublining. Thermal conductivity is low and thus the material gives good protection against thermal stimuli applied to metallic restorations.

Glass-ionomer (polyalkenoate) Type III lining materials are particularly suitable where cariostatic action is required, although there are reports that pulpal inflammation is produced when used in deep cavities. Where dentine is less than 0.5 mm thick, calcium hydroxide should therefore be used as a sub-base. These lining materials adhere to tooth substance and are suitable as a structural base.

Calcium hydroxide can neutralise free phosphoric acid of phosphate cements and the pH of 11–12 prevents the survival of microorganisms found in carious dentine. Besides being a pulp capping agent, calcium hydroxide is employed in deep cavities prior to the placement of a structural base. It can also used to protect the pulp under composite material, provided there is no solvent in the formula as this may plasticise some resins. Some calcium hydroxide materials are considered too weak to allow condensation of amalgam without the additional placement of a structural base.

15 (a) This lady is suffering from a local hypersensitivity reaction to rubber. Rubber gloves were worn during an examination procedure for an edentulous patient whose mandible was manipulated to achieve the retruded arc of closure. Interestingly, there were no intra-oral lesions. Following the occurrence, the patient gave a history of having previously developed an allergy to rubber while working as a kitchen assistant washing dishes. She should be reassured that the local irritant effect of the rubber will resolve spontaneously in due course.
(b) Obviously, rubber gloves should not be worn and vinyl examination gloves could be substituted. At the same time, other rubber-containing products should not be used on the patient; i.e. polysulphide impression material. Likewise, although of irrelevance in this case because the patient was edentulous, rubber dam could not be employed during endodontic therapy for a dentate patient giving a similar history. It is unclear whether synthetic rubbers (i.e. silicone rubber impression materials) should be avoided.

16 (a) This radiographic view is called a bitewing and it will have been taken to assist in the diagnosis of occlusal and approximal caries.
(b) Each film has a 'blip' on it, with a convexity on one side and a concavity on the other.

When the film is exposed the convexity faces the tube. The film should be mounted and read on an illuminated viewing box with this convexity facing towards the person reading the film.

(c) The radiograph shows occlusal caries in the upper and lower first molars. There are no approximal lesions apparent. (Compare the radiographic appearance of the first molar tooth with the clinical view, *Figure 2*.)

(d) The approximal surfaces of these teeth appear superimposed. This may have occurred because the teeth in this area are imbricated, causing overlapping of the contact points on the film. This overlapping makes the diagnosis of approximal lesions in enamel difficult.

(e) The radiolucent shadow on the mesial aspect of the upper first molar is the cervical radiolucency, not dental caries. Cervical radiolucency is a normal appearance and is caused by the absence of the dense enamel cap at the cemento-enamel junction and the absence of the interdental alveolar bone.

17 Incomplete coronal fractures can be detected by:

- *Visual inspection* following careful drying of the tooth. Good lighting is essential and the use of magnification may be helpful.
- *Transillumination.* This may reveal a fracture as a dark line or as a line of transition where the intense light is prevented from further entry into the tooth by the fracture.
- *Dyes.* Following the removal of a restoration from a suspect tooth, the application of a dye solution (e.g. ink, disclosing solution, food dye) may enable a hairline fracture to be seen more readily.
- *Wedging.* Patients should be asked to bite on a small solid object (e.g. cotton bud, rubber wheel, golf tee) placed in relation to individual cusps of the suspect tooth. Pain may be elicited on clenching or on release of pressure due to the opening and closure of the fracture.
- *Percussion of individual cusps.* Percussion or the application of gentle pressure to individual cusps may elicit pain or precipitate complete fracture of the affected cusp.
- *Radiographs.* Periapical radiographs rarely allow clear visualisation of vertical coronal fractures unless the plane of fracture coincides exactly with the plane of the radiograph or the fragments are well separated.

18 (a) The most likely cause for the continual dislodgement of the post crown is the short wide preparation that is clearly visible. In addition, occlusal interferences in protrusion and lateral excursions may be contributing factors.

(b)
- The dimensions of the post hole make it mandatory that the root should be carefully examined for a vertical fracture. Indeed, whenever a post repeatedly debonds this should be undertaken. It is best achieved by inserting an instrument into the post hole and gently leaning it towards the periphery. This has the effect of opening the fracture, should one exist. The pressure applied should not be such that it precipitates a fracture!
- A periapical radiograph should be taken in order to determine the length of root available to receive a new post. This will also confirm the apical status of the root as well as indicating if any obstruction in the canal, e.g. fractured post or instrument, would prevent an adequate depth hole being prepared.
- The occlusion should be carefully assessed to ensure that interferences in excursive movements are not a dislodging influence.

(c) If the root has a vertical fracture it will require extraction with subsequent replacement by a temporary partial denture. When healing has occurred the mouth should be fully assessed to determine the suitability for a permanent fixed or removable replacement.

If the root is intact an attempt should be made to lengthen the canal preparation, taking care not to perforate the root. The most appropriate method for gutta-percha removal is the range of Gates Glidden[1] burs, which are non-endcutting and therefore follow only the path of the GP. Ideally, the depth of the post hole should be approximately equal to the length of crown to be replaced but it should be recognised that this will vary with individual clinical circumstances. Once an adequate depth has been achieved, the canal should be widened to appropriate dimensions. With the size of post hole illustrated, it would be prudent to bevel the root face in order that a cast diaphragm can be used as a ferrule to prevent subsequent root fracture.

If the canal is blocked and it is not thought possible to increase the depth of the preparation then some other form of core construction should be considered; e.g. a pinned composite or amalgam. However, the amount of available root face for the insertion of the necessary pins is restricted and if a perforation occurs the root will again require extraction with subsequent prosthetic replacement.

Occlusal interferences will require adjustment. This may involve the simple incisal reduction of an overerupted lower incisor or more substantial equilibration. It may be necessary to consider constructing the post and crown as a single casting if space is severely limited.

19 (a) Either transfer copings or occlusal registration copings.
(b) They may be used for:
• Localisation of dies from different impressions.
• Checking the accuracy of dies.
• Occlusal registration for articulation.

Impressions. When taking an impression of several preparations, it may not always be possible to achieve a perfect reproduction of every one. Retaking the whole impression might be successful but a useful technique is to make dies of the satisfactory preparations and construct transfer copings on these. At the patient's next visit the copings are tried on the preparations; this will give a good indication of the quality of the dies. The preparations that were missed in the first impression can be isolated with the copings left in place on the preparations already satisfactorily recorded and a new impression taken. The existing dies are replaced into the copings (removed within the new impression) and a new model poured. There will therefore be dies from the first impression localised alongside and in the correct relationship to dies from the second impression.

Occlusal registration. The most accurate way of localising two opposing models is to avoid any form of interocclusal record and place them together in the most favourable interlocking position—the position of best fit—and compare them with the patient's intercuspal position. This avoids the inaccuracies of the common wax 'squash bite'. However, where there are several preparations or where teeth are missing, such a position of best fit may not be found. In this case, provided the patient still has some teeth determining the vertical dimension, the most accurate record will be made by fitting copings, which are just clear of the occlusion, and adding fresh acrylic to their surfaces prior to asking the patient to close the teeth together. When set, the copings will provide a rigid and accurate record for articulation.
(c) The usual material for coping construction is an acrylic resin with good colour contrast, such as Duralay[2] or Palavit G[3]. They are made on a die produced from the preliminary impression and their margins should be trimmed carefully to those reproduced on the die. The coronal contour should be shaped to allow accurate pick-up in the secondary impression if their use is intended for this purpose.

20 (a) The tentative diagnosis is a dental abscess of pulpal or periodontal origin. To make a definitive diagnosis, the lower incisors and canines should be examined for suggestions of pulpal necrosis due to extensive caries, large restoration or physical trauma. Identification of a non-vital tooth or teeth by some form of pulp test would be needed to confirm the diagnosis. If all teeth proved to have vital pulps, then a periodontal examination would be necessary to discover a periodontal abscess or extensive pocket. This would be aided by the use of periodontal probes and periapical radiographs. The identification of the path of a periodontal pocket could be assisted by the insertion of a radiopaque marker, such as a GP point, prior to taking the radiograph.

(b) If acute, confirmed by high temperature and pulse, antibiotics should be given. Drainage should be established as soon as possible by incision of the external abscess when this proves to be fluctuant. If the definitive diagnosis indicates a pulpal origin, drainage of the pulp chamber of the tooth or teeth involved via the cingulum region should be obtained.

21 (a) The patient has a parafunctional habit and the associated tooth-wear has caused a number of working side and non-working side interferences to manifest. These have stressed the posterior restorations and teeth leading to restoration failure.

(b) The cast restorations have been based on a diagnostic wax-up. Their purpose is to provide canine guidance with posterior disclusion during mandibular movements. The effect of this will be to exert less lateral stress on the posterior restorations and cusps. It may be necessary to provide the patient with a protective splint to be worn at night if restoration failure occurs due to continued bruxism.

22 (a) Acrylic resin is used where strength is required for thin patterns that are to be removed from a working cast. The material is, however, subject to contraction and distortion prior to investment and casting and this will result in a metal framework which does not fit. Any errors may go unnoticed when the restoration is tried in the mouth and will result in an excessively thick resin lute, the bond strength of which reduces with increased thickness.

(b) Distortion of large spans may be minimised by waxing patterns directly onto a refractory die, thus avoiding the requirement to remove the pattern before investing. This reduces distortion of the castings to a minimum.

(c) If a pattern is not removed from a working cast there is no opportunity to check if margins are extended into undercut areas. When cast in metal these will prevent accurate seating unless they are removed. The finished casting must be carefully tried on a master stone model and undercuts removed before further processing. Waxing directly on to a refractory investment limits the methods of retention that may be used for the metal. The technique works best with full-coverage retainers cast in non-precious alloy where retention to resin is provided either by grit blasting and chemical adhesion, or by gel/electrolytic etching with acids.

23 The use of a low-viscosity intermediary resin reduces the risk of marginal gap formation and marginal discoloration. Many in-vitro bond strength investigations have revealed no significant difference between the bond strength of composite resin to acid-etched enamel, whether an intermediary resin has been used or not. However, these were conducted under ideal laboratory conditions and involved the application of the composite resin to a small flat enamel surface. Clinical trials (Hansen *et al.,* 1984) reveal an increased incidence of marginal discolorations and marginal gaps when intermediary resin is not used before composite resin application to Class III, IV and V acid-etched cavities.

24 (a) Gold can be surface-treated in three ways to render it adhesive to chemically active bonding resins.
• *Application of a pyrogenic coating* with a Silicoater[4]. This technique deposits a thin layer of silicon oxides onto the surface of the gold in a high-temperature environment. The layer acts as a coupling agent between the metal surface and the resin luting cement.

- *Tin plating.* A tin-plated gold surface will have a stable tin oxide layer on its surface to which chemically adhesive resins can bind.
- *Oxidising the surface.* Gold alloys containing greater than 8% copper can be oxidised at 400°C in air for 10 min to form a stable metal oxide layer on the surface of the alloy. This too will give a stable bond to resin luting agents.

(b) *Gold* is the least damaging of the three materials. It is easy to adjust in the mouth and can be finished to a high lustre after finishing, if that is appropriate. It is somewhat ductile in nature and this is thought to minimise damage to opposing tooth structure.

Non-precious metals are very hard and tend to be difficult to adjust and polish in the mouth. In addition, the casting accuracy of non-precious alloys is less than that for their precious counterparts. Non-precious alloys will tend to cause relatively more damage to the opposing tooth tissue, but can be used reliably in thinner sections than gold.

Porcelain is difficult to construct to give an accurate occlusal scheme. If adjustment is necessary after cementation, the adjusted surface cannot be reglazed and will tend to be rough, producing accelerated wear of the opposing tooth tissue. Adjusted porcelain surfaces will tend to accumulate more plaque than glazed porcelain surfaces.

(c) Cast gold is best polished to a high gloss followed by sandblasting the occlusal/contact surfaces with a 40 μm alumina. This surface will be easier to mark with articulating paper, or in function if temporarily cemented, than a highly polished surface, and can be easily polished back to a high shine if that is preferred by the patient.

25 (a) While the detail produced in a condensation silicone impression is satisfactory for advanced operative work, the dimensional changes which occur, particularly with the light-bodied materials, can result in difficulties in the placement of the final restoration. This can be overcome by having a very thin film of light-bodied material supported by the very much more dimensionally stable putty.

(b) The two-stage technique was originally developed to offset the rapid setting of the impression materials. By manipulating only one material at any one time the operation was simplified. To achieve success it is essential that adequate venting of the putty impression is carried out, otherwise the light-bodied material will pool within the primary impression. The putty itself is rigid when set and it is wise to ensure that it has been relieved to provide a loose fit. This can be achieved with a spacer and the added bulk of the more elastic light-bodied material enables the dies to be removed from the impression without fracture.

(c) There are some limitations of this technique:
- Failure to wash the putty adequately can result in separation of the two phases of the impression.
- Inadequate reseating of the tray or uneven pressure during the second stage can result in an incorrect occlusal relationship with the adjacent and opposing teeth.

26 (a) To facilitate micro-mechanical resin bonding to the retainer wing.

(b) The surface treatments, which may be carried out to facilitate metal–resin bonding, can be classified as follows:
- Macro-mechanical, which relies on visible undercuts, usually with perforated metal, pitted metal or a wire mesh.
- Micro-mechanical retention, which is dependent on microscopic porosities such as sandblasting and etching.
- Interfacial bonding, which may also be used by placing a secondary interface on the metal surface to which a composite resin may be attached; i.e. silicoating or tin plating.

(c) The original luting cements for resin-bonded frameworks were basically microfilled composite resins, such as Comspan[5]. More recently, resin–metal adhesives have been introduced—e.g. Panavia Ex[6], Superbond[7] and, most recently, All-Bond 2[8].

27 (a) The upper left lateral incisor shows gingival recession.

(b) The anterior teeth have all been restored with porcelain veneers. No tooth preparation was undertaken and after cementation the operator failed to remove all the excess luting composite resin from the cervical region of the left lateral veneer, resulting in plaque retention and gingival irritation, which has led to the recession.

Damage to the marginal gingivae during:
- tooth preparation
- gingival retraction for impression taking
- isolation of the tooth during cementation
- removal of excess luting resin
- finishing of the cervical margin of the cemented veneer
- reduction of the bulk/contour of the porcelain margin

may all encourage gingival recession, particularly if the gingival condition is unhealthy before restoration or if there is an underlying dehiscence or alveolar deficiency. Excess luting cement may be difficult to identify and remove during finishing/polishing after cementation because it may match the existing tooth colour very closely and be bonded to tooth enamel beyond the veneer margins after acid-etching of this region.

(c) The treatment that was required for this patient was simply removal of the excess luting resin, and the marginal gingiva returned to its original position within 2 weeks. Patients should always be recalled within a week or two of cementation of a veneer to check for excess luting composite.

28 Zinc phosphate luting cement has been in use for many decades and has been relatively successful. It has the thinnest cement film thickness of any luting cement. Its disadvantages are that it has no adhesive properties and there is anxiety about its low pH in the unset state.

Alternatively, glass-ionomer (polyalkenoate) luting cement has the advantage that it exhibits some chemical adhesion to the prepared tooth. It has the added advantage that it has the potential to assist in preventing caries at the margin of the cemented crown by fluoride release and, after the initial setting period, it has a lower solubility than zinc phosphate cement. Its disadvantage is that it has a higher cement film thickness than zinc phosphate cement.

29 (a) It is important that the restoration is coated with a water-resistant layer as soon as possible. At this early stage many Ca^{2+} and Al^{3+} ions will not have reacted with the poly-alkenoate and may be washed out, preventing the full set of the material. Also, much of the water in the material is still unbound. If the restoration dries out at this early stage, it is likely to craze on the surface.

(b) Ideally, the restoration should be coated with a layer of unfilled polymer resin, such as a fissure sealant or enamel bonding resin. Alternatively, one or two layers of cavity varnish may be applied.

(c) This should be delayed for at least 24 h to allow adequate strength to develop.

(d) They are directly adhesive to the calcified dental tissues without the need for an intermediary bonding system.

(e)
- Type I luting materials have very small glass particles containing radiopaque ions such as strontium.
- Type II reinforced materials contain small amounts of silver and are commonly called cermets (ceramic metals). They are the most radiopaque and least aesthetic of the GPA cements.
- Type III lining materials have larger glass particles than the luting materials, with relatively high amounts of fluoride to decrease the setting time. The glasses are also radiopaque.

30 (a) The tooth is being prepared so that a sealant restoration (sometimes called a preventive resin restoration or PRR) can be placed.

(b) This type of restoration combines caries removal and composite resin restoration with sealing of the remaining fissure system.

(c) A rubber dam is being used because isolation from saliva is important in order to obtain a good physical bond between the enamel and resin via the acid-etch technique.

(d) The surface of the enamel appears 'frosted'. This has been achieved by the application of phosphoric acid, which has been used to etch the enamel in order to provide retention for the composite restoration.

(e) The white material in the base of the cavity is a proprietary lining material that contains calcium hydroxide. It is used to protect the dentine from the effect of the enamel etchant. Materials containing eugenol are unsuitable as they will have a plasticizing effect on the composite resin and prevent complete polymerisation.

31 Management options for the tooth include:

Extract. Advantage—simple approach, particularly if no prosthetic replacement is necessary. Disadvantages—may result in tooth drifting, loss of masticatory function and compromised aesthetics if space not restored. A fixed prosthesis would be damaging to abutment teeth, while a removable prosthesis may be poorly tolerated and compromise dental health.

Hemisection with extraction of buccal roots; root-canal therapy and crown to restore palatal root. Advantage—relatively simple root-canal therapy, only one root to restore. Disadvantages—the poor alignment of the palatal root in the dental arch compromises the aesthetic result of the final restoration.

Hemisection with extraction of the palatal root; root-canal therapy and crown to restore the buccal roots. Advantage—the excellent arch alignment of buccal roots does not compromise the aesthetic result. Disadvantages—root-canal therapy and restoration of two buccal canals is more complex. Extraction of the palatal root may be difficult due to path of withdrawal. Bony resorption may lead to a furcal periodontal lesion between buccal roots.

32 (a) The material is being mixed by an operator wearing gloves.

(b) Sulphur compounds within the latex (acting as a surfactant and accelerator) act as a catalytic poison on the platinic acid catalyst of the impression material. This, therefore, retards the set of the material, and the resultant impression will be distorted, with a poor surface finish, and be unsuitable for model construction.

(c) To prevent this problem, gloves should be removed and hands washed to eliminate any residual sulphur compounds before mixing. Alternatively, an auto-mix cartridge system or vinyl gloves, which are free from contaminants, may be used.

33 (a)
- The patient should be asked why the teeth were crowned and what they were like initially (are any photographs available?).
- It should be determined when tooth movement was first noticed.
- Any contributory habits should be identified.
- An analysis of the occlusion may be necessary.
- An assessment of the periodontal status should be undertaken.

(b) The most likely cause for the tooth movement is that the previously proclined teeth have now been placed in an unstable position, with the lips being unable to counteract the action of the tongue. In addition, the lower lip may catch the incisors and act in a manner similar to an orthodontic appliance. This will be of special relevance if the crowns have been made too long. Finally, there is the possibility that a previously undiagnosed periodontal condition has reduced the bone support of these teeth.

(c) The proclining teeth could be retracted if it is assessed that there is sufficient bone support. Linked crowns should be constructed to act as a permanent splint and care taken with the design of their length and palatal contours so that there is correct incisal guidance. This can be assisted with the aid of diagnostic waxings. As an alternative to a permanent splint, a night appliance could be considered.

34 (a) Non-working side contact or interference.
(b) The clinical significance is controversial. In the early literature on occlusion, which was then the province of the prosthetists, the non-working side was referred to as the balancing side and the non-working interference shown would have been called a balancing side contact. This reflects the tooth arrangements required for complete denture base stability.

It is now believed that there should be no tooth contacts on the non-working side and that the spatial position of the mandible should be determined by the non-working condyle on the one side and the tooth contacts on the other. Some workers consider non-working contacts to be of no significance, provided there is no evidence of TMJ/muscle dysfunction. However, others believe strongly (it must be said, in the absence of any scientific evidence) that such a contact is an aetiological agent for TMJ/muscle dysfunction syndrome and that it should be corrected by occlusal equilibration.

The more practical aspect is that if a crown preparation is to be undertaken on a tooth involved in such a contact, then the occlusal reduction involved in the preparation might simply equilibrate the arrangement, allowing the non-working condyle to take up its proper position on the articular slope, which would be more superior. This would mean that when the preparation was examined in lateral excursion, there would be no apparent occlusal reduction.

In this case, the relationship should be equilibrated prior to the crown preparation.

35 (a) There is an isthmus fracture of the amalgam restoration, severing the box portion from the retentive keyway. Although the amalgam box is still *in situ,* the marginal seal around it will have broken, thus allowing seepage and the development of caries.
(b) Essentially, the cause is a weakness of the amalgam in the isthmus region. The width of the isthmus seems adequate and the maximum that can safely be obtained for a tooth of this size. The weakness, therefore, is probably because the amalgam is too thin, either because the cavity was shallow or its base/lining was too thick. Other possible causes could be that cervical recurrent caries has eliminated the 'resistance form' supporting the box and allowed it to flex and fracture, or the patient could have bitten heavily on the newly placed amalgam, thus causing fracture before it had fully set and hardened. Alternatively, the restoration may have caused interference with the opposing teeth, but there is no evidence here of a 'high spot'. The restoration could have been satisfactory when originally placed but received some excessive occlusal force from a hard item of food or a blow to the mandible.
(c) The action required to replace the amalgam restoration with one having a good prognosis depends upon the cause of the fracture. If this was due to isthmus weakness, strength must be obtained by ensuring adequate thickness in the amalgam, use of amalgam with good strength properties maximised by thorough condensation and the avoidance of moisture contamination which would weaken the amalgam. The restoration must be carved to avoid interferences and the patient warned to avoid chewing on the filling until it is fully set. It is, of course, mandatory that all peripheral caries must be rigorously removed to prevent further recurrence.

36 Three groups of tooth-coloured materials are currently available for restoring cavities in this position: composite resin; glass-ionomer (polyalkenoate) cement; and the new copolymer visible light cured glass-ionomer hybrid materials.

- Composite resin will bond securely to enamel and dentine with appropriate treatments. Fully polymerised composite, which has aged or been instrumented, bonds poorly to new resin and would provide minimal adhesion to the replacement bridge.
- Glass-ionomer cement bonds securely to tooth tissues and to composite resin but lacks the aesthetic qualities required for the labial surface of the restoration.

The best solution would be to place glass-ionomer cement in the palatal part of the restoration to the full depth of the cavity to provide support to the bridge in this region. The remaining labial part of the cavity, which will not be covered by the bridge, can be restored with composite resin bonded to the underlying glass-ionomer and surrounding enamel.

37 (a)
- Internal bleaching and replacement of palatal amalgams with composite resin restorations
- Porcelain or composite resin labial veneers with or without the addition of internal bleaching
- Post-crown restorations.

(b) *Internal bleaching* and restoration with composite restorations may provide an acceptable appearance provided the discoloration is related to pulp death of the teeth and not the result of amalgam-corrosion products penetrating the dentine. It is a relatively non-invasive procedure but there is a tendency for any lightening effect brought about by the bleaching to regress with time. *Porcelain* or *composite veneers* do require some reduction of labial enamel and involve the placement of a restoration margin adjacent to the labial gingival margin but they are much less destructive than post or jacket preparations. Use may be made of opaque cements to complete the camouflage of the underlying discoloured tooth substance.

The provision of *post-crown restorations* would involve the loss of significant amounts of coronal and radicular dentine, thus making the tooth weaker and more prone to root fracture. It also involves the replacement of the natural tooth crown with an artificial substitute. It is a more predictably successful treatment than jacket crowns, the preparations of which are not generally recommended on root-filled anterior teeth. Access cavity and root-canal preparation involves the removal of much coronal dentine, which is normally relied upon to provide the core for a jacket-crown preparation.

38 (a) The most reliable predictors of caries activity are texture and degree of dampness of the suspect tissue. Soft/crumbly wet dentine is most likely to be active; dry firm tissue is likely to be arrested. Colour is *not* an accurate predictor of disease activity. Texture should probably be monitored using the side of a sharp excavator to prevent a probe from creating an uncleansable defect in the surface of the root, which would lead to disease progression.

(b) An alteration in the oral environment either associated with an increased frequency of dietary sugar intake or an alteration in salivary function.

(c) Management would obviously depend upon both the aetiology and the extent of the caries. If diet was the principal factor involved, then appropriate dietary advice should be given, including the substitution of fermentable carbohydrate with other sweetening agents (diabetic sweets, sugar-free chewing gum, etc.) where possible. Alterations in salivary flow are managed by a variety of strategies covered in Answer **10**.

Management of the carious lesions would depend upon their depth and extent:
- Shallow lesions are amenable to remineralisation using a combination of topical fluorides, either professionally applied or as a daily rinse, chlorhexidine mouthwash and supersaturated calcium phosphate mouthrinses. Initial therapy should be relatively aggressive, with regular professional topical fluoride applications. Maintenance therapy would include the regular use of a fluoride mouthrinse and dentifrice.

- Deeper lesions (0.5–1 mm) can be managed by recontouring the surface using fine abrasives, followed by the same active prevention/remineralisation regimes outlined above. Both of these approaches will result in the production of arrested lesions that are hard, but tend to be darkly stained.
- Finally, more extensive lesions can be restored, preferably using a glass-ionomer (polyalkenoate) cement.

(d) Lifelong residence in a community with a fluoridated water supply results in a reduction in both the prevalence and severity of root-surface caries. In addition, a topical effect with reductions in both prevalence and severity has been demonstrated for adults who live for protracted periods (more than 30 years) in a fluoridated community.

39 (a) Following radiographic examination to determine the root morphology and that there is no other local trauma, the pulp should be extirpated under local anaesthesia and arrangements made to initiate root-canal therapy in order to obtain a good apical seal. If local soft-tissue damage has occurred and the fractured fragment cannot be accounted for, further radiographic views will be necessary to eliminate its impaction into a wound.
(b) Surgery to the palatal soft tissue will expose the margin of the tooth. This will, however, produce a rather irregular gingival contour which will predispose to periodontal problems. An alternative approach would be to extrude the tooth orthodontically which, although extending the period of treatment, will maintain the gingival contour.
(c) Exposure of the margin is essential in order that it can be satisfactorily recorded in an impression. This will enable the final crown margin to have an acceptable marginal fit and not initiate gingival irritation.

40 (a) Several factors have probably contributed to the unusual pattern of loss of tooth substance in these lower molars. Slowly progressing carious lesions, as indicated by the degree of staining of the dentine, is the most likely initiating factor, followed by fracture of undermined cusps. The exposure of the underlying dentine would then make the teeth more susceptible to the effects of erosive and abrasive elements of the diet. The original position of the pulp chamber, now filled in with reparative dentine, can clearly be seen and indicates the chronic nature of tooth-substance loss.
(b) The main difficulty in restoring these teeth will be the limited height of the clinical crown and the lack of retention that can be provided for any restoration that is attempted. In addition, although not shown in the illustration, there is also likely to be a lack of interocclusal clearance because of the over-eruption of the opposing teeth.
(c) Full veneer crown restorations or adhesive onlays would be suitable treatment options, once sufficient interocclusal space had been created following adjustment of the opposing teeth. If crowns were to be placed, crown lengthening may be required to increase the height and surface area of the preparation.

41 (a) CAD/CAM stands for computer-aided design/computer aided-manufacture, techniques that are common in industry. Used initially for the repetitive manufacture of precision items, CAD/CAM techniques have more recently been developed to produce one-off items. In dentistry, a number of systems are being developed and the inlay shown in *Figure 38* was manufactured using the Cerec[9] system, which is already commercially available, although expensive.
(b) The limitations are that the only available systems to date can produce only a limited range of restorations, and they are very expensive. However, the same was true of computers only a decade or so ago and it is likely that CAD/CAM techniques will increasingly find a role in operative dentistry.

42 (a) The margins show the effect known as ditching.

(b) Two main processes contribute to this phenomenon:

• First, as a result of occlusal forces at occlusal contact areas, the amalgam is subject to creep and the material at the periphery flows upwards to protrude above the enamel margin. These unsupported edges of amalgam subsequently fracture, leaving a ditch. This process is exaggerated if the amalgam margin angle is too acute.

• Secondly, corrosion in the marginal interface may contribute to the gap.

(c) No, the marginal ditches are not usually carious and are sealed at their depth by corrosion products. Obviously, active recurrent decay requires treatment.

(d) Condensation of the amalgam ensures maximum adaptation of the amalgam to the cavity wall and eliminates excess mercury. This increases the strength of the set material, thereby reducing the potential for creep. It also minimises the formation of the γ_2-phase and, consequently, corrosion.

43 (a) As the restoration involves the incisal edge, the tooth should be restored with a composite, as glass-ionomer (polyalkenoate) cements do not have sufficient fracture resistance in this situation.

(b) Although there is some mechanical retention, this must be supplemented with a dentine and enamel bonding system.

(c) No. Provided there is sufficient reactionary dentine, it is possible to bond the composite to dentine with a dentine bonding system. However, if there is any leakage of the restoration, or a trans-dentine exudation of pulpal tissue fluid, then the bonded composite would not be cariostatic. In this situation, a glass-ionomer lining will leach fluoride and reduce the likelihood of recurrent decay.

(d) Within reasonable limits the working time is controlled by the dentist. It can be relatively long for a large restoration or short for a simple case. However, once activated, a working initial set is formed very quickly.

44 (a) The occlusal surface of the lower second premolar shows an occlusal carious cavity and a white spot lesion on the fissure walls. A student failed to observe the lesion because the tooth was examined wet and a bubble of saliva covered the fissure system.

(b) A bitewing radiograph is required before treating the tooth operatively, so that the dentist can see whether there is an approximal lesion. The radiograph did in fact show a large occlusal lesion in the dentine. Since lesions are larger clinically than they appear radiographically, it is possible that the pulp was exposed. It would therefore also be necessary to perform a vitality test since pulpal necrosis could have occurred, necessitating root treatment. In addition, therefore, a periapical radiograph should be taken and examined for periapical radiolucency. If root-canal treatment is necessary, this radiograph can be used to check root canal morphology before starting the operative procedure.

45 (a) Thermal pulp vitality testing with heat. A heated gutta-percha stick is applied to a moist or Vaseline-coated tooth.

(b) Application of heat to a tooth with an irreversibly inflamed pulp would be expected to elicit a painful response, which persists following the removal of the heat source. Thermal vitality tests should always be interpreted with caution and, where possible, more than one test of vitality should be undertaken.

46 (a) This material, which sets to a rubbery consistency, allows temporary cementation of cast or porcelain restorations. In this way the fit, appearance and function of the restoration can be assessed. Further occlusal adjustments prior to final cementation can also be carried out.

(b) For bridge cementation, the rubber-like quality allows minor realignment of the preparations during trial cementation. This will not happen with other materials which are non-elastic. A zinc oxide/eugenol cement mixed with petroleum jelly or Tempbond[10] with a modifier may be used, but neither of these is as easily removed from the fitting surfaces of restorations. Neither Tempbond[10] without modifier nor a thin mix of zinc oxide/eugenol should be used as a trial cement because, due to their thin film thickness, it may prove impossible to remove the 'trial' cemented restoration for final placement.

47 (a)
- A full dental examination to identify the number of teeth affected by the condition.
- An assessment of any habits or dietary intake which might be contributing to the wear pattern.
- Vitality testing of the involved teeth.
- Measurement of the resting lower face height to determine the freeway space.
- The construction of a diagnostic overlay to assess the possibility of permanent encroachment on the freeway space in order to re-establish the lower face height.

(b) In order for crowns to be constructed for the upper anterior teeth, interocclusal space will need to be created. For this to occur, the patient must be able to tolerate an increase in the lower face height so that lost tooth tissue can be replaced with crowns.

If space is achieved with a removable overlay appliance, a night guard will be required to prevent all the occlusal forces being transmitted to the newly crowned teeth when the overlay is removed at night. Alternatively, the new face height could be maintained by crowns in the posterior quadrants. This, however, is a substantial undertaking and is unlikely to be justified.

If the worn teeth are found to be non-vital or if it is considered that their reduced clinical height will jeopardise the retention of the crowns, thought will have to be given to devitalising the teeth and the subsequent construction of post retained crowns.

If no increase in face height can be tolerated a decision may have to be made to replace the teeth by means of an overdenture or, alternatively, simply to counsel the patient to accept the inevitable continued loss of tooth substance.

48 (a) A deprogramming jig for occlusal registration.

(b) The manipulation of the mandible by the operator on to the retruded arc of closure is an essential part of the technique for the registration of centric jaw relation. Some patients may subconsciously resist this manipulation, showing a preference to use their habitual arc of closure into centric occlusion (intercuspal position).

The memory of the centric occlusion position is short term, lasting only about 10 min, provided the teeth do not touch in that time. The deprogramming jig may be made at the chairside for resistant patients and prevents tooth contact for the appropriate period. After this time, the operator repeats the manipulation, which should then be effective.

49 (a) Enamel hypoplasia, resulting from disturbance of the enamel matrix formation by some systemic cause such as an exanthematous fever in childhood.

(b) Yes, the hypoplasia is linear and thus time-related, as indicated by the fact that the areas affected would have been expected to be forming during the same period of the dentition's development. In this example of a permanent dentition, the tips of the upper incisors are hypoplastic whereas in the lower incisors the hypoplasia involves a band of enamel 1 mm below the normal incisal tip. The lower teeth tend to develop slightly ahead of the upper teeth and the pattern shown here is consistent with a disturbance occurring at the age of 2–3 years.

(c) It is unlikely that there are any symptoms from this degree of hypoplasia.
- If the patient is young and unconcerned about the appearance, it may not be necessary to intervene for a few years, unless it is predicted that the absence of upper incisal tips may lead to disfiguring over-eruption.

- If appearance is of concern, the deficiencies of enamel could be restored with acid-etched composite. Retention, however, which depends on the existence of normally calcified enamel for the formation of retentive tags, could be a problem with the upper incisors. Tips of acid-etched composite would have to be extended onto sound enamel, both labially and palatally.
- A better solution would be the use of porcelain veneers or, if the patient is of the age to ensure maturity of the gingivae and pulp size, the use of jacket crowns could be considered.
- The defects in the lower incisors are surrounded by normal enamel, and composite restorations could be etched to these successfully and with minimum interference.

50 (a) The post has been made too short to provide adequate retention in the first instance. Following debonding, food debris and saliva enter the root-canal preparation and coat the walls with bacterial plaque. This is difficult to remove successfully before recementation, because adequate instrumentation risks widening the post hole. In addition, a poor cementing technique may produce air voids in the canal space, reducing support to the post.
(b) All plaque, debris and old cement must be removed from the retainer and the preparation.
- The retainer may be grit-blasted or ultrasonically cleaned.
- The preparation should be carefully inspected for signs of old cement. Fine spiral brushes driven by a slow-running handpiece can be used to scrub the walls of a post hole with pumice and conventional brushes used to clean other types of preparation. Mechanical instrumentation with twist drill or burs will remove tooth tissue, increase cement thickness and weaken the cement lute.
Failure to remove all the old cement will prevent correct seating, produce increased cement thickness at the margins and cause occlusal interference.
- Adhesive luting agents improve retention above that of conventional luting cements.
- Luting agents should be placed carefully to avoid inclusion of air.
(c) This post crown has been grit-blasted with 50 μm particles to remove debris and clean the surface. A simple chairside electroplating unit is applying tin diethylenetriamine solution, carried in a porous anode tip, to the fitting surface of the post crown. The plating circuit is completed by connecting the cathode to the polished metal surface of the crown. A thin, firmly attached layer of tin is deposited on the fitting surface. Plating must take place within 15 min of grit-blasting to obtain the best result.
(d) Most resin bonding agents do not bond well to precious and semi-precious alloys. Tin plating deposits a layer of non-precious metal on the surface which oxidises on exposure to air and bonds strongly to chemically adhesive resins, such as Panavia Ex[6]. Adhesion of resins which do not chemically bond to non-precious metals is facilitated by first coating the tin-plated surface with a metal primer such as 4-META. A dentine bonding agent must be used to bond the luting resin to the preparation.

51 (a)
- The crown of the premolar will have been weakened by the development of caries and the subsequent cavity preparation required for the MOD amalgam restoration.
- There is evidence of a non-working side interference on the amalgam surface.
- Over-eruption of the tooth or the antagonist may have occurred as a result of the restoration having been carved initially out of occlusion. Premature contact between the weakened palatal cusp of the tooth and the opposing tooth cusp in the presence of parafunctional activity may have led to cusp fracture.
(b) Pain due to thermal and osmotic stimuli as a result of exposed dentine.
(c) Temporary restoration could involve the placement of glass-ionomer cement after cleaning the exposed tooth surface with polyacrylic acid and resurfacing the adjacent

amalgam with a diamond bur. For a more permanent result, thought should be given to placing a pinned amalgam core, followed by the construction of a three-quarter gold or metal–ceramic crown.

52 (a) The surface of the cement has become dehydrated during the placement procedure or during finishing. This chalky appearance is characteristic of such dehydration and may be associated with cracking of the surface of the cement. This is more of a problem when multiple restorations are placed under a rubber dam, when great caution must be exercised to prevent excessive drying of the cement after removal of any surface matrix.
(b) The appearance of the material will improve with time, as the water balance improves within the cement as a result of exposure to the oral environment. The first task would be to persuade the patient to leave things alone for a while to see what improvements occur with maturation of the cement. If the patient remains dissatisfied, it may be necessary to replace the restoration using another shade of glass-ionomer (polyalkenoate) cement or a composite resin. Placing a surface veneer of composite over this restorative-grade material is a possibility, but it may cause future diagnostic dilemmas as the cement is radiolucent (see Answer **163**).
(c) The best surface finish for a glass-ionomer cement is that obtained against a surface matrix: either cellulose acetate, mylar or aluminium.

Upon removal of the matrix at the completion of the setting reaction for the cement, the surface of the restoration should be protected from early desiccation/moisture contamination by the use of a barrier varnish (*not* copal–ether varnish as this permits the rapid diffusion of water), cocoa butter or, preferably, by the placement of a thin layer of unfilled composite resin-bonding agent on the surface of the cement. This will form a minimally permeable barrier of BIS-GMA/urethane diacrylate resin on the surface of the cement, which provides the greatest duration of protection for any of the methods mentioned.

Placement of the varnish/resin on a partially set cement surface will result in an excessively rough surface, which should be avoided if possible.

Surface finishing of glass-ionomer cements should be limited to removal of gross overhangs and other major errors at the initial placement visit. The surface of the cement should then be varnished and the material allowed to mature fully prior to definitive finishing at a review appointment.

Definitive finishing can be achieved using Arkansas stones with a petroleum jelly lubricant, or mounted aluminium oxide abrasive discs. Care should be taken to avoid excessive heating of the cement surface as this will cause disruption of the hydrogel matrix of the set cement. Finishing discs should be lubricated with either petroleum jelly or with water during these procedures.

53 (a) The combination of metal and ceramic provides both the strength required for this type of restoration and the aesthetics which the patient desires.
(b) In all cases the use of a metal occlusal surface is preferred to ceramic as there is a risk of considerable damage to the opposing tooth tissue when the latter is used. This is particularly the case where adjustments of the occlusal surface are carried out at the fitting stage and the ceramic is not reglazed. It is also much easier to reproduce acceptable occlusal morphology using the lost wax technique than by shaping porcelain.
(c) There are three cements which may be suitable, although they all have their limitations:
- *Zinc phosphate cement* is considered by many to be the cause of pulpal trauma following crown cementation and it will only mechanically interlock with the irregularities of both the fit surface of the crown and tooth preparation.
- *Zinc polycarboxylate cement* will adhere to dentine but has a long elastic-setting phase. It initially leaches fluoride.

- *Glass-ionomer (polyalkenoate) cements* adhere not only to dentine but also to suitably treated metals. Type I luting glass-ionomer cements have been reported to cause pulpal irritation in a limited number of cases. They do, however, release fluoride ions over extended periods of time.

(d) Tooth preparation for metal–ceramic crowns requires substantially greater tooth tissue removal in order that there can be sufficient thickness of ceramic and metal to provide both strength and satisfactory aesthetics. A shoulder width of 1.5 mm will therefore be necessary. Occlusal reduction will be dependent on whether the restoration will be of metal or ceramic/metal in this area. If the latter, again a reduction to allow 1.5 mm thickness of materials will be required. Ceramic crowns need a minimum overall reduction of 1 mm to give the crown sufficient strength, while all-metal crowns should allow occlusal coverage with at least 1 mm of metal—but, cervically, this can be thinned to a knife edge and thus be more conservative of tooth tissue.

54 (a) The platinum or palladium foil matrices.

(b) These should have been removed prior to cementation of the crowns. In the case of jacket crowns they are *in situ* during their construction only to serve as a matrix to prevent the unfired porcelain from 'slumping' when the crown build-up is removed from the die and in the firing process.

(c) In the McLean/Sced technique, twin foils are employed: one foil, after being tin plated, is fired as an integral part of the core; the second foil is removed in the traditional manner.

(d) This type of crown is said to impart strength to the restoration, as it prevents the propagation of microcracks. At the same time maximum aesthetics are imparted to the crown because it has no metal core preventing transmission of light. The tin plating of the inner foil aids the physico-chemical bonding that can be achieved with adhesive luting materials.

55 (a) The upper incisor teeth are short although the labial surfaces appear not to have changed in shape. The lower incisor teeth have over-erupted to meet the upper incisors. Bulimia nervosa is the condition in which patients (often young and female, but not exclusively either) develop bizarre eating habits, including episodes of deliberate vomiting to remove food bulk. Some bulimic patients vomit several times per day. The effect of this is to produce rapid palatal erosion of the upper incisor and premolar teeth and sometimes of other tooth surfaces as well. In the case shown in *Figure 54*, the palatal surfaces were badly eroded and the incisal edges had also been lost. The lower incisor teeth were much less affected, which is typical of the condition.

(b) The patient is likely to complain of the appearance of her anterior teeth but not usually of sensitivity. It will often be difficult to elicit the history of bulimia nervosa but this presenting condition is so typical that the possibility should always be investigated.

(c) When the appearance is not badly affected it is better to try to defer treatment until the condition becomes less acute. Often, patients revert to normal eating habits after a few years of a bulimic eating pattern. However, in a case as severe as this, treatment to improve the appearance of the upper incisor teeth can also help the patient to develop a greater sense of self-respect and can contribute to their general health and in some cases may indeed be contributory to overcoming the bulimia. The ideal solution here would be to depress the lower incisor teeth by a removable orthodontic appliance or by a cemented Dahl type of appliance. Once this is done the upper teeth can be prepared for crowns without preparing the incisal edges or the palatal surfaces any more. In this case retention was possible without additional retentive means. Sometimes crown lengthening is carried out to improve retention, but in this case this would have produced an unrealistically high gingival contour and was not necessary.

56 (a) The position of the gingival margin of an *amalgam restoration* is dictated primarily by the extent of the carious lesion. Black's concept of extension for prevention, whereby cavities were extended subgingivally, has been shown to lead to periodontal disease rather than to have any effect on the prevention of caries. In the case of approximal boxes the gingival margin should clear the contact area to allow adequate finishing of enamel margins and placement of a matrix band.

(b) Likewise, with *composite restorations*, the shape of the cavity is dictated primarily by the shape of the carious lesion. It is preferable to retain the gingival margin in enamel if this is possible in order to bond the composite to the etched enamel. If the caries extends on to the cementum, the use of a glass-ionomer laminate technique or dentine bonding system is recommended to seal the restoration and prevent microleakage.

(c) Prior to preparing any tooth for an *extracoronal restoration*, all caries should have been removed and the tooth restored with a suitable core material. The following factors will, therefore, influence the position of the finishing line:

- *Aesthetics.* The margin of an anterior crown would normally be placed at or just into the gingival crevice for the best appearance.
- *Substructure.* Where aesthetics is not an important consideration, the gingival margins of extracoronal restorations should be placed supra-gingivally. Ideally, this should be on sound tooth substance or amalgam. If the core material is glass-ionomer (polyalkenoate) cement or composite, the preparation should be extended sub-gingivally in order that this may be achieved.
- *Retention.* Along with factors such as degree of taper and surface area of the preparation, the height of the preparation is an important parameter with regard to retention. In cases of short clinical crowns, the margin of the crown may necessitate sub-gingival placement to increase the effective length of the preparation.

57 (a) First, root dentine is more susceptible to caries than is enamel. Also, setting contraction tends to pull the composite away from the cavity walls. This shrinkage is resisted by any adhesive bonds to the cavity margin. In the case shown in *Figure 55*, good adhesion was attained to the enamel margin and therefore the contraction forces pulled the setting composite away from the dentine margin. Recurrent caries has developed in the resulting gap.

(b) Provided the patient was satisfied with the appearance of the restoration, the cervical caries could be removed, leaving the coronal composite in place. The base of the cavity should be explored to eliminate the presence of undermining caries and then the inset filled with composite together with a dentine bonding agent or, alternatively, a glass-ionomer (polyalkenoate) filling.

(c) A dentine bonding agent should be used to reduce the chance of cervical leakage. The cavity should be packed with small increments of composite, starting at the dentine margin. The increments may be of varying shade to match the tooth.

58 (a)

- A rubber dam is being used to exclude saliva from the cavity, thus aiding vision and preventing moisture contamination that adversely affects any of the materials subsequently used to restore the tooth.
- The exclusion of moisture will also prevent contamination of the pulp should the tooth be exposed during cavity preparation.
- The application of a rubber dam also helps to retract the cheeks and tongue, thus making operating easier.

(b) Having gained access to the caries, a round bur should be used to render the enamel–dentine junction caries-free. This area is said to be clinically caries-free when it feels hard to a sharp probe and is stain-free.

(c) When the enamel–dentine junction has been cleared, a sharp excavator should be used to remove all soft caries from the pulpal surface of the cavity. Stained but firm dentine should be left to avoid a pulpal exposure.

(d) If a carious exposure is found, pulp extirpation and root-canal therapy will probably be required if the tooth is to be saved. A small exposure, surrounded by firm dentine, may occasionally be pulp-capped with a proprietary setting cement containing calcium hydroxide if the tooth is symptom-less and vital, the object being to induce dentine bridge formation and preserve pulp vitality.

59 (a)
  (i)   A dental panoramic tomograph.
  (ii) Right and left bitewings.
  (iii) Periapical radiographs of potential abutment teeth; root-filled teeth; heavily restored or crowned teeth, where doubt exists of their vitality; symptomatic teeth which may require endodontic treatment.

(b) *A dental panoramic tomograph* provides general information relating to the teeth and supporting structures as well as the position of unerupted teeth, retained roots and bony pathology.

   Bitewings give more precise details of:
• The anatomy of the enamel, dentine and pulp chamber.
• Site and extent of carious lesions and exisiting restorations.
• Contact relationships of teeth and presence of overhanging cervical margins and the fit of inlays and crowns.
• Interdental bone levels.
• Presence of both supra- and sub-gingival calculus.
   Periapical radiographs are to provide details of:
• The supporting structures of teeth and root-canal anatomy.
• The existence of root fractures.
• Height and quality of bone support.
• Width of the periodontal ligament space and integrity of lamina dura.
• Presence of bony pathology related to the teeth.
• While also of use in the diagnosis of caries, a less-distorted image will be provided by a bitewing and these should be used in preference—although distortion can be reduced by the use of the long cone paralleling technique.

60 (a) The veneers are of a single shade, while the surrounding teeth exhibit banding due to tetracycline staining. Furthermore, the veneers are large, with a poor labial contour, which is not in harmony with the patient's natural teeth. The shade selection of the veneers is also incorrect.

(b)
• An attempt to lighten the patient's natural teeth with bleaching should be carried out to disguise the subtle banding. This will probably make the existing veneers more obvious but they should not be replaced until the degree of lightening of the other teeth is determined so that they can be matched more easily.
• If bleaching fails to improve the appearance of the other teeth or replacement of the veneers still does not result in a satisfactory appearance, the veneering of at least 321│123 will probably be necessary to provide a reasonable appearance.
• Depending upon the patient's smile line, the premolars may also require veneers.
• To assess fully the appearance before proceeding, it is advisable to produce a diagnostic wax-up of the proposed treatment. This will allow both the operator and patient to judge

the effect of altering the relative size of the teeth. The wax-up will also provide the technician with a guide to veneer construction.
- Opaque porcelain and luting cement will probably be required to mask the tetracycline staining.

61 (a) A dentine screw inserted into the canal of the tooth.
(b)
- Difficulty in removing the existing root filling to create space for the screw.
- Perforation of the root by the use of an incorrect instrument.
- Insufficient clinical crown height to 'house' the screw head and to provide an adequate bulk of restorative material.
- Disturbance of the endodontic seal.
- Fracture of the root during placement.
(c)
- Cast post/core.
- Cemented stainless steel post.
- Pinned core.
- Amalgam slots.

62 (a) There is over-eruption of the upper first permanent molar into the space left by the extraction of the lower molar.
(b)
- The normal history and examination should include vitality tests and periapical radiographs of the over-erupted tooth and of the teeth either side of the lower space. With the agreement of the patient, the lower molar should be replaced to stabilise the occlusion. The complicating factor is the over-eruption, which will compromise the construction of a prosthesis and introduce occlusal interferences.
- The first stage is to correct the occlusal plane by providing a crown on the upper molar after removing the existing amalgam and checking the structure of the tooth and its biological state. In this case, the tooth was vital and a pinned amalgam core was provided, followed by a metal–ceramic crown.
- The lower arch could be restored by means of a partial denture, particularly if there were missing teeth on the opposite side, a conventional bridge or a resin-retained bridge. Given the excellent condition of the abutment teeth and the remainder of the mouth, the resin-retained bridge is the preferred option.
(c) Possible consequences of leaving the condition untreated include:
- Drift of teeth either side of the space with tilting and opening of associated contact points with food packing and gingivitis. The former, in turn, could lead to approximal surface caries.
- The tilted teeth may lead to the development of deflecting occlusal contacts.
- The final consequence can already be seen; i.e. the over-eruption of the opposing tooth.

63 (a) This is a bitewing radiograph and will have been taken to assist caries diagnosis. A clinical examination appeared to show the teeth to be caries-free. The radiograph also shows the level of alveolar bone and can be used to assess the extent of interdental periodontal destruction.
(b) The lower first molar has a mesio-occlusal metal filling. A radiolucency is present in the dentine beneath the occlusal aspect of the restoration. This represents carious demineralisation and the tooth should be treated operatively.
(c) The lower second premolar shows a distal carious cavity that extends through the enamel and into the dentine. This tooth should also be treated operatively.

(d) The upper first molar has an occlusal metal filling. The radiolucent area in the outer enamel is dental caries which may be arrested by preventive treatment. This should include diet analysis and advice, flossing the contact to remove plaque and the use of fluoride-containing toothpaste. Another radiograph should be taken in a year to monitor caries control. In a patient with multiple carious lesions, preventive treatment should always accompany operative treatment.

64 (a) Dye has penetrated along the gingival floor and up the axial wall of the cavity preparation. The dye has travelled along a gap formed between the restoration and the tooth from the external gingival margin, indicating a bond failure in this region. Gap formation extending this far provides a pathway for toxins and possibly bacteria to contaminate dentine close to the pulp. Pulpal inflammation will occur and secondary caries may develop on the gingival floor. Post-operative pain and sensitivity are attributed to this phenomenon.
(b) The primary problem with direct composite restorations is polymerisation shrinkage, which may be up to 2% in volume. This contraction produces tensile stress around the walls of the cavity preparation. Debonding will occur in areas of weakness and a gap develops as the strain in the resin is released. The weakest area in posterior proximal restorations is along gingival floors, where the enamel is thin and etches with a type III amorphous pattern, giving relatively little mechanical bonding to the resin. The tensile bond strengths of current dentine bonding systems are not sufficient to resist polymerisation contraction forces and significant debonding occurs in this critical region. The resin bond is further stressed in the mouth by differential thermal expansion and contraction and by mechanical stress from the opposing teeth. Light activation of composite resin from the occlusal surface results in resin contraction away from the inner surfaces of the preparation before it has polymerised.
(c) Composite resin with high filler loading will contract the least during polymerisation. It is important to apply the resin in increments to distribute stress and to guarantee its full polymerisation. The technique which produces the least experimental leakage involves placing a small increment of resin in the floor of the box and curing with the aid of light-conducting wedges to initiate polymerisation from the tooth/resin interface. Further larger increments are placed on the vertical walls and cured from the adjacent buccal or lingual side. This method ensures shrinkage towards the preparation surface. If a cavity is large, it is more appropriate to use indirect restorations, such as composite or ceramic inlays/onlays, where the problem of polymerisation contraction is largely eliminated.

65 (a) A major difficulty for any technician is to determine the cuspal movements of the dentition using hand-held casts or casts mounted on a simple hinge articulator. The functionally generated pathway technique allows these movements to be recorded in wax intra-orally and transferred to the articulator in the form of a static plaster cast (the functional index). By registering the pathways of the opposing tooth surfaces during mandibular movements, the technique allows a laboratory technician to provide a restoration with an occlusal surface less likely to incorporate occlusal interferences.
(b) The involved tooth should be immobile and the recording material retained on the prepared tooth, not moving separately, during the generation of the FGP wax record. The involved tooth should have unprepared teeth anterior and posterior to it to act as reference surfaces for checking the complete seating of the functional core on the working cast. There should be no occlusal interferences pre-operatively and the opposing occlusal surfaces should be satisfactorily restored.

66 (a) The margins of the restorations are standing proud of the surrounding tooth tissue. Assuming that the restorations were well adapted originally, there appears to have been loss of either tooth tissue or luting material from the margins of the restorations.

(b) Question the patient about oral hygiene and dietary habits, and attempt to ascertain the type of luting cement used to attach the restorations to the tooth surface in the first instance.
(c) Differential diagnosis:
• *Loss of luting agent from the margins of the castings.* A possibility, although the marginal defects are rather large for this to be the sole cause. The cement could simply have washed out if a relatively soluble material had been used (i.e. zinc oxide/eugenol or zinc poly-carboxylate) or have been dissolved via plaque or dietary acids.
• *Loss of tooth tissue through oral hygiene.* An unlikely cause of this localised destruction. There is little evidence of loss of tooth tissue further towards the cervical margins of the teeth.
• *Loss of tooth tissue through acid dissolution of the tooth substance.* The most likely cause of this appearance, with a regurgitation-type of acidic exposure just extending onto the buccal surface of the upper teeth.
(d) This patient had bulimia, which had not been controlled. An attempt had been made to restore teeth using adhesively retained metal shims on the palatal surfaces of the upper arch. Continued acid dissolution of the marginal tooth tissue has occurred, resulting in marginal ditching, with the development of extensive carious lesions beneath the restorations. Such restorations should not be placed in the presence of recurring acid.

67 (a) The cavity has been prepared with no regard to modern principles of cavity preparation.
• The occlusal key was almost certainly unnecessary, as there is no evidence of caries at the base of the fissure.
• The key is excessively wide but has not been cut into dentine.
• With regard to the interproximal preparation, this has been extended excessively bucco-palatally, and bears little resemblance to the shape of the original carious lesion.
• The cavo-surface angles are in excess of 130° rather than at 90°, the angle required for amalgam preparations.
• Marked trauma of the gingival tissue is present on the palatal side as a result of careless use of rotary instruments.
(b) If an amalgam restoration were to be placed in the cavity, bulk fracture of the amalgam would most probably occur at the junction of the isthmus and approximal box due to inadequate thickness of amalgam. Buccal and palatal marginal fracture of the amalgam is also likely because of the thin margins of amalgam, which are a consequence of incorrect cavity preparation in these areas.

68 Recent developments in the understanding of caries pathology have led to an understanding of the dynamic nature of the caries process, with the capability of many incipient lesions to undergo remineralisation if the environment is favourable. Traditionally, sharp dental probes have been the key tools in caries diagnosis, detecting roughened areas of early enamel breakdown on smooth surfaces and 'stickiness' or resistance to withdrawal following their forceful insertion into suspect pits and fissures. It is now clear that the use of sharp probes in this manner may often be detrimental, causing frank cavitation of previously intact surfaces with a change in the local environment inconsistent with arrest and remineralisation of the lesion. It is generally recommended that the current role of the dental probe in caries diagnosis is one of a cleaning device to allow better visualisation of the surface being examined. In order to avoid damage to the surface of the incipient lesion, it is recommended that probes should be blunted for use in this cleaning role.

69 The following features should be examined to determine the reasons preventing the satisfactory fit of the bridge:
- The cast and preparations, to ensure that there are no undercuts to a communal path of insertion/withdrawal.
- That there is no temporary cement remaining on either abutment tooth, especially in the depth of any retentive grooves.
- The presence of tight proximal contacts.
- Over-extension of margin(s).
- That the tissue surface of the pontic is not causing gingival blanching.

If the bridge fails to seat fully or does so only with sustained firm pressure which, when released, allows the bridge to spring off the anterior abutment, then the problem is likely to be one of incorrect location of the retainers and/or tooth movement due to inadequate or lost temporary restorations. A non-setting cement may be used (e.g. zinc oxide/eugenol mixed with Vaseline) or a silicone-based proprietary material, such as Opotow Trial Cement[11], for a few hours to allow the teeth to realign themselves within the retainers.

If this does not succeed then the bridge should be sectioned between the pontic and the distal retainer. If both retainers subsequently seat fully they require re-location with plaster (or with zinc oxide/eugenol or Duralay[2] resin) intra-orally. Wax is added to the index to stabilise the relocated bridge units, to create a mould space for the solder assembly and to protect the porcelain. The units are invested and after setting the wax is eliminated and the connector joint soldered. If the bridge still fails to seat, a new impression will be required to enable it to be remade.

70 (a) A midline diastema might be the result of:
- Small teeth in a large or normal-sized upper jaw.
- Missing lateral incisors.
- Unerupted canines, with or without the retention of the deciduous predecessors.
- A persistent labial frenum.
- The presence of a mesiodens, supplementary or supernumerary tooth or other midline pathology.
- Periodontal disease.
- A habit.

(b) The possible effects of operative intervention could be demonstrated to the patient by any of the following techniques:
- The teeth to be involved, either the central incisors alone or in conjunction with the lateral incisors, could be prepared on a model and restored with laboratory-made acrylic crowns eliminating the diastema. If the patient decides to proceed with the treatment these crowns can be used as temporary restorations while the new crowns are being made.
- If only the central incisors are to be restored, a small fillet of acrylic, or a diagnostic wax-up with ivory wax, can be made to eliminate the space. The former can be tried-in at the chairside but both very effectively demonstrate to the patient the effect of space elimination.
- Similarly, the mesial surfaces of the incisors can be prepared for the placement of acid-etched retained composite restorations to alter the contours of the teeth. The result achieved may be sufficient to satisfy the patient's demands without having to resort to more substantial treatment.
- Still using composite resin, veneers can be constructed and placed on the teeth with a non-curing medium. It should be explained to the patient that the appearance will be bulkier than that eventually achieved because there has been no tooth reduction.
- Less satisfactory, but still giving visual impact, is the careful retouching of a photograph.

(c) It is important that patients are given some idea of the effect of operative treatment;

otherwise, there is a possibility that, on completion, they may express their disappointment and declare that if they had realised how their appearance would be changed they would have stayed as they were!

71 (a) This restoration has been incorrectly contoured, resulting in a flash of composite overhanging the labial margin. As this part of the enamel was not etched, oral fluids have penetrated beneath the flash.

(b) Correct contouring of restorations to avoid thin overhanging flashes.

(c)
- Microfilled composites consisting of pre-polymerised polymer–colloidal silica complexes embedded in a polymer matrix reinforced with further colloidal silica particles.
- Hybrid composites consisting of glass particles embedded in a polymer matrix reinforced with colloidal silica.

(d) Because all of the filler particles in the microfilled materials are smaller than the wavelength of visible light, they retain the ability to reflect light despite surface wear.

(e) The shiny surface indicates that this is probably a microfilled material.

72 (a) Perforation into the furcation area by a tapered screw post intended for the molar's distal root.

(b) The operator obviously lost the line of direction due to carelessness; this was possibly compounded by the lack of a pre-operative radiograph and obscured vision due to the presence of a rubber dam. The roots are filled with silver points which, if not removed, would be impossible to reduce in length in order to make access for the screw post: the reamer will be deflected laterally by the silver. If it can be anticipated that a screw post will be required at some time in the future, then root canals should be filled with gutta-percha or, in exceptional circumstances, with an apical-section silver point to avoid this problem.

(c) Furcation involvements usually mean a very poor prognosis for the tooth. If the bone was only minimally damaged by the reamer and the post was sterile, the situation may resolve without symptoms developing—but this must be regarded as optimistic. If not, then the choice is between extraction probably followed by a fixed–fixed bridge to prevent the lower second molar from tilting or hemisection with the placement of a full crown on the mesial root.

73 (a) Electrical pulp vitality testing.

(b)
- A conductive medium should be applied to the test tooth to ensure good current flow through the tooth.
- The test tooth should be isolated from adjacent teeth to prevent current passing to neighbouring teeth, thereby producing erroneous results.
- Patients should contact the metal surface of the electrode in order to complete the electrical circuit required for the test to function. Contact between an ungloved hand of the clinician and the mucosa of the patient is no longer acceptable practice in the current climate of cross-infection control.

74 (a) A crown-retained, fixed–movable bridge.

(b) In function, a fixed–fixed bridge would transmit much of the force onto the cement lute retaining the post in the canine, causing it to fail. However, as the bridge is also retained by the central incisor, the bridge could remain *in situ,* with the failure of the post element undetected. A real possibility then exists that caries may develop in the root face and post hole of the canine. The provision of a movable component will produce a 'stress broken' effect. Forces will be placed on the post retainer in a more favourable manner, and cement lute failure should be less likely. However, if failure does occur, looseness, or loss, of the bridge should aid early discovery, thus enabling caries to be prevented from destroying the abutment tooth.

(c) Provision of a simple cantilever bridge using the canine as the sole retainer could be considered. A separate crown on the central incisor would be necessary only if clinically indicated. Care, however, should be taken during fabrication of the bridge to ensure that the pontic is only contacted in the intercuspal position and discludes during any mandibular movements. The retainer on the canine should, preferably, be constructed to provide group function rather than canine guidance during lateral excursions. This will avoid undue stress being transferred to the radicular dentine via the post. It would be unnecessary to use both the canine and first premolar as abutments to replace the lateral. There is also no indication for placing a spring cantilever bridge in this case.

75 (a) The restoration has failed because the post has fractured within the canal.

(b) An attempt should be made to remove the fractured post element. The most suitable method is to trephine the dentine surrounding the post. The Masserann[12] kit (Micromega) provides a range of hollow-end cutting burs which remove a narrow band of dentine from around the post in order to allow the insertion of a tighter-fitting bur which is used to extract the retained post (or fractured instrument). When such a kit is unavailable it may be possible to drill into the post if it is made of yellow gold and subsequent vibrations may loosen it, thus allowing it to be retrieved. An ultrasonic instrument may, likewise, break the cement lute.

(c) If it is not possible to re-establish the post hole, it will be necessary to construct a pin-retained core in either a composite material or amalgam. Specific coloured composite core materials are available to allow easy differentiation between dentine and core.

76 (a) The bridge replacing the upper first premolar shows extremely poor technical work. There are areas of thin or perforated ceramic which are poorly glazed, no palatal cusp on the pontic and metal subframe showing which is not intentional, i.e. it has been revealed after adjusting the ceramic to accommodate the occlusion. The mesio-occlusal amalgam in the molar is grooved, presumably by careless crown preparation.

(b)
- The poorly glazed ceramic may abrade the opposing teeth as this surface is composed of rough particles of considerably higher surface hardness than enamel.
- The failure to provide a centric stop for the opposing lower canine has led to its over-eruption, i.e. there has been loss of occlusal stability. The lower tooth became aesthetically unacceptable to the patient, which led him to seek treatment. This involved orthodontics to realign the over-erupted tooth followed by the remaking of the bridge to provide a centric stop. With the new bridge the opportunity should be taken to ensure that the occlusal relationships are correct so that no chairside adjustments are necessary.
- The grooved amalgam may lead to food packing in the poor contact area and should, therefore, be replaced.

77 (a) The palatal cusp has fractured due to lateral stresses from mastication or possibly due to an interfering occlusion. The fracture was made more likely by the extent of the MOD cavity.

(b) It may have been prevented if the tip of the palatal cusp had been reduced to take it out of lateral excursion contact with the opposing cusp. If the original caries had been minimal and confined to the mesial and distal surfaces, excessive weakening of the tooth could have been prevented by the use of independent self-retentive box restorations. If the size of the MOD cavity could not have been kept smaller, then support for the remaining tooth tissue could have been obtained by restoration with an acid-etched retained composite, a capped-cusp inlay or a full-coverage crown.

(c) Unless it is already known that the tooth is root filled it should be tested for vitality. The fractured cusp will require removal to determine the level of fracture and in order that this can be accomplished the palatal tissue requires anaesthetising. It may be necessary to incise the gingival cuff so that the fragment can be removed without traumatising the soft tissue. If the fracture line is below the bone level this will indicate that the tooth should be extracted, as it will not be possible to create a satisfactory finishing line for a restoration. If less extensive, a temporary repair could be achieved with glass-ionomer (polyalkenoate) cement. A more permanent solution will necessitate the removal of the existing amalgam and the placement of a pinned retained core followed by a cast restoration to protect the remaining cusp. It may be necessary to root-fill the tooth, in which case some form of post/core restoration may be thought to be more appropriate.

78 (a) Intracoronal restorations are not normally recommended as major retainers for bridges. They do not provide enough retention and resistance when secured with conventional luting cements because they fail to distribute applied forces over the entire preparation surface and are unable to withstand tensile loading. Metal inlays are sometimes used with resin-bonded bridges but the metal is extended to the preparation margins. In this case the metal component is a substructure covered with ceramic extending to the margins. The ceramic forms a large part of the fitting surface.

(b) This design of bridge must be cemented with a composite resin using appropriate agents to promote bonds between the luting resin, and enamel, dentine, ceramic and metal. A nickel chrome metal substructure is the main tensile load-bearing component which has a very high elastic modulus, rendering great stiffness to the bridge. This is enhanced by the very high modulus of the bonded ceramic. The substructure is cast from a conventional wax pattern. The finished casting is placed on a duplicate refractory die onto which ceramic is added. The refractory material is bead-blasted from the fitting surface, which is then etched with hydrofluoric acid, rendering it highly retentive to composite resins. A tooth-coloured, dual-cure resin of the correct shade is used to bond the bridge. This produces an almost invisible junction between the enamel and ceramic surfaces and gives an excellent aesthetic result. Stress from applied loads is distributed via the resin to the entire fitting surface of the abutment preparations.

(c) Partial or full veneer crowns could be used as major retainers, in a fixed–fixed design, with the possibility of an inlay as a minor retainer in a fixed–movable design. Core restorations would be required as part of the treatment. Conventional designs have a long history of success but are destructive of tooth substance and give poor aesthetics where laboratory work is not of the best quality. Metal wing retainers extending lingually could be used to support a resin-bonded, minimal-preparation bridge design. The existing amalgam restorations would, however, need replacing with glass-ionomer (polyalkenoate) cement as composite resin bonds less well to amalgam. Posterior minimal-preparation, resin-bonded bridges are not as successful as their conventional counterparts and optimal designs will expose metal on the buccal aspect of the abutments. The present design conserves tooth tissue by utilising the existing space of the previous cavity preparations.

79 (a)
- The restoration in the upper left central incisor appears dark throughout its bulk.
- The Class IV restoration in the upper right incisor shows evidence of both cervical marginal discoloration and surface discoloration. There would also seem to be surface wear, with a loss of contour and surface reflectivity.

(b)
- The left tooth has been restored with a chemically activated composite which has darkened as a result of amine discoloration.
- The composite restoration in the right incisor is light-activated material and the cervical discoloration could be due either to unbonded cavo surface marginal excess retained as a 'flash' or inadequate isolation of the region between etching and bonding.
- The surface discoloration is due to porosity caused by entrapped air.
- The loss of reflectivity will be caused by resin matrix abrasion with subsequent filler particle loss, which leads to a rougher surface.

(c) The Class III restoration in the left central incisor could be replaced totally with a modern colour-stable light-activated composite resin restoration employing the acid-etch technique to aid retention and marginal integrity. The restoration in the right incisor could be veneered with a layer of microfilled or sub-micron (polishable) hybrid composite after reducing the surface of the old filling to roughen it and expose a 'fresh' surface for bonding. Any cervical marginal excess should be removed and the adjoining enamel etched (after rubber dam isolation) before applying intermediary resin and new composite.

80 (a) Loss of vitality of the upper left central incisor with associated pulpal necrosis and dentine discoloration.

(b)
- Vitality tests.
- Radiographs.

(c) The treatment strategy would involve:
- Providing adequate endodontic treatment for the tooth in the first instance.
  Complications. The complications for this phase of care could include an old root fracture making endodontic treatment difficult and, possibly, sclerosis of the root canal.
- Subsequent to endodontic treatment, non-vital bleaching could be attempted to improve the colour of the tooth. (See Answer **95**). Ideally the tooth should be taken a shade lighter than the surrounding teeth as there will be a tendency for the colour to relapse with time.
  Complications. Non-vital bleaching is a viable option only with adequate endodontic treatment. It is not always successful and no reliable predictors of success are available. There is a tendency for relapse.
- The other treatment options include the use of surface veneers of composite resin or porcelain, or a full coronal restoration.
  Complications. Masking a severe discoloration with a veneer can be difficult without producing an excessively bulky restoration. Colour matching against an adjacent natural tooth is also difficult when using a surface veneer approach.

81 (a) Gingival retraction, in this case using an Epipak[13] ring.

(b) Gingival retraction is required to expose the margins of crown preparations which are placed at or below the gingival crest. This retraction is necessary to allow an accurate impression of these areas to be recorded.

(c)
- Mechanical retraction using suture silk may be used where gingival health is excellent and minimal retraction is required.
- More commonly, a combination of mechanical and chemical retraction is employed with cords impregnated either with a vasoconstrictor, such as adrenaline, or astringent, such as aluminium chloride. In addition to the mechanical displacement provided by the cord, chemicals are incorporated to produce tissue-shrinkage and to control haemorrhage and crevicular seepage. If the cord can be placed below the margin of the preparation, it should be left *in situ* during the impression stage. Alternatively, two fine cords may be placed, the

outer one being removed immediately prior to injecting the impression material into the gingival sulcus.

Retraction with impregnated cords causes trauma and induces inflammation to the epithelium of the sulcus and underlying tissues. However, provided careful techniques are employed, there should be no clinically significant changes in healthy gingival tissues. Several authors feel however that, in view of the potential systemic effects which may arise from the use of adrenaline-soaked cords, these should no longer be used.

- Electrocautery may be used to form a trough around the preparations by removing tissue from the wall of the gingival sulcus. Great care must be employed when using this instrument, as potential exists for serious damage to the periodontal ligament and surrounding bone, resulting in loss of attachment of the tooth. The equipment must not be used on or in the vicinity of patients with cardiac pacemakers.

82 (a) There is a mesio-occluso-distal restoration of a densely radiopaque material, probably cast metal. Between this and a radiopaque layer over the dentine, there is a discrete and regular radiolucent void.

(b)

- The tooth may have had a restoration placed over a radiolucent cement; for example, Type II glass-ionomer (polyalkenoate) cement.
- Alternatively, there could be a cement void following cementation of an inlay with an inadequate amount of cement.
- It may be that a base material was removed simultaneously with a temporary dressing and, as the inlay margins were well-fitting, the void was not apparent clinically.

The appearance is unlikely to be due to secondary or residual caries because the shape of the radiolucency is regular and well demarcated.

(c)

- The treatment option, if the use of a radiolucent base was recorded, would be to monitor the radiographic appearance and intervene only if the area was getting larger on sequential radiographs.
- If no record of the base material is available, or you suspect 'cement starvation', a decision to intervene should be made on the basis of the integrity of the restoration margins.
- If the restoration margin is poorly adapted, removal and replacement of the restoration is required; otherwise, recurrent caries may affect the deep dentine surfaces of the cavity.
- If the restoration appears to be well-fitting, efforts to remove the inlay should be made; these should, however, fall short of irreversibly damaging the restoration. If the inlay can be removed easily, the base material (if present) can be inspected and the inlay recemented with an adequate amount of cement. If the inlay cannot be easily removed the area should again be monitored with the use of sequential bitewing radiographs.

83 (a) A provisional restoration should restore both the form and function of the tooth or teeth. The materials used in their construction should be:

- Non-irritant to the underlying pulp or the surrounding gingival tissue.
- Aesthetic, especially if placed in the anterior parts of the mouth.
- Strong in thin section and capable of withstanding occlusal forces for a reasonable period of time.
- Low in thermal diffusivity.
- Easy to manipulate if the restorations are to be made at the chairside.
- Low in setting dimensional change.
- Limited in exothermic reaction if cured intra-orally.

(b) While the resin-based materials used in the construction of provisional restorations provide a means of temporarily restoring teeth they cannot be relied upon to maintain adequate occlusal stability. They exhibit considerable wear and the possibility exists that occlusal surfaces will perforate. Besides jeopardising tooth position, especially if there is gross loss of material, exposed dentine may become sensitive.

(c) Non-precious metal and acrylic-faced metal restorations should be constructed in cases where there is loss of a substantial component of the occlusal table during bridge and crown preparation in order to avoid these occurrences.

84 (a) Two types of defect can be noted on the model:
- Voids in the stone resulting from a poor casting technique, where air incorporated in the plaster during mixing has not been removed by vibration during the casting process.
- Finer voids present on the palatal surface of the incisor teeth. These have been caused by hydrogen bubbles produced during the setting of the impression. The polymerisation mechanism of the impression material is by addition-crosslinking, catalysed by a platinum catalyst, which theoretically does not produce any by-products. The hydrogen bubbles are the result of impurities, such as small-chain polymers with hydroxyl groups.

(b) Any cast restoration constructed on such a model would have a poor marginal fit as a result of irregularities incorporated into the margins of the castings because of the voids in the stone model.

(c) It is recommended that addition-cured silicone impressions are left for 1 h or longer before pouring stone casts. Other methods include subjecting the impressions to a vacuum either before or after pouring the casts.

85 (a) There is little or sometimes no enamel present in this region for bonding. When present, the enamel may be aprismatic, which is not ideal for etching.

(b) It is essential to use a dentine bonding agent to attain good adhesion to the whole cervical floor. The composite should be packed in oblique increments to prevent the polymerisation contraction pulling the material away from the floor.

(c) Light-curing materials contract towards the activating light. If the materials are activated from the occlusal direction, then the material contracts towards the light and away from the margin, resulting in a cervical gap. The refractive wedge transmits light to the cervical margin and activates polymerisation at this site. The resulting contraction is therefore towards the free surface of the composite and not the cervical margin.

86 (a) The gums are red and swollen and there are heavy deposits of plaque on the cervical margins of the teeth.

(b) The gums will bleed when a periodontal probe is used because the epithelial lining to the gingival sulcus has increased vascularity and is friable and therefore easily traumatised.

(c) The enamel around the gingival margins consists of white patches which are white spot lesions—early enamel caries.

(d) This patient has both gingivitis and dental caries. Preventive treatment is required and its success will depend on the patient's cooperation. The patient came to your surgery aware of the gum problem and is therefore likely to do their best to improve the oral hygiene under your tuition. With good cleaning, resolution should be quite rapid and if the patient has been shown the red, swollen appearance of inflammation they will see the gums change colour, texture and contour. You will have to explain the significance of the white spot lesions and how these can be arrested by a change of diet, improved cleaning and sensible use of fluoride. A diet sheet will help you to give advice on the cause of dental decay and how the diet could be modified. Improved plaque control, with a fluoride-containing toothpaste, will also help to prevent further demineralisation. This patient will need constant encouragement and careful monitoring.

87 Routine application of a rubber dam during operative procedures may be advantageous both to the operator and patient by providing:

- *Moisture control.* This is critical to the successful outcome of many operative dental procedures, notably those involving the bonding of restorative materials to tooth tissue and those involving the handling of materials whose physical properties may be significantly compromised by moisture incorporation (e.g. amalgam). The prevention of contamination by the microflora contained in oral fluids is also central to the success of pulp-capping and endodontic procedures.
- *Protection of the patient* against damage to the oral tissues by irritant or toxic materials and against the loss of materials and instruments into the oropharynx.
- *Protection of the dentist* and supporting personnel against cross-infection by significantly reducing the levels of microbe-laden aerosol, which are generated during high-speed cutting procedures.
- *Improved visibility* for the practitioner by retracting soft tissues and providing good colour contrast with the teeth under treatment.
- *Improved patient comfort* by allowing patients to isolate themselves from operative procedures, which are effectively being undertaken outside their mouths.

88 The tooth pictured has had a Nordin[14] screw placed in the root-canal system. If the tooth were decoronated prior to core placement, there would be little resistance to torsional forces acting upon the screw post. The result of this would be that the post may unscrew during function, with subsequent failure of the core and crown. If tooth substance is retained, the placed core will prevent torsional forces acting directly upon the post; i.e. an anti-rotational device will be incorporated. Additional benefits conferred by the retention of tooth substance include:

- The possibility of a more robust preparation.
- Greater freedom in choosing the position of the crown margin compared with preparing a previously decoronated and cored tooth.
- Increased retention for an adhesive cermet core if this material was selected to replace missing tooth substance.

89 (a) The patient's main concern is likely to be related to the presence of the midline diastema. However, she may also dislike the prominence of the pointed canines, which are made more noticeable by the absence of lateral incisors.

- The simplest form of treatment would be for the pointedness of the canines to be camouflaged by the application of acid-etched retained composite in conjunction with slight grinding of the tips of the teeth. A reduction in the width of the diastema could also be achieved by the addition of composite to the mesial surfaces of the central incisors.
- Alternatively, if the patient was prepared to undergo a course of orthodontic treatment, space could be created for the prosthetic replacement of the missing lateral incisors by closure of the diastema and retraction of the canines by means of a fixed appliance. Additional space may need to be created in both upper quadrants by the extraction of teeth. Once tooth movement is complete, the lateral incisors should be replaced with a removable denture or minimal-preparation bridges. Later, thought could be given to the construction of fixed–fixed or cantilever bridges if considered appropriate.

(b) Both treatments could be commenced immediately but the construction of permanent bridges should be delayed until the patient is about 20, so that the gingival margins are stable and the pulp chambers of suitable dimensions.

90 (a)
- Marginal staining.
- Recurrent caries under the palatal cusp of the first premolar.
- Poor approximal contact.
- Poor marginal adaptation of the approximal material in the second premolar.

(b) These faults are typical of poorly placed posterior composites which have been present some years. They are the result of a combination of clinical placement errors and difficulties with deficiencies in the material properties.

Clinical placement
- The placement of a posterior composite is time-consuming and is far more difficult than the placement of the equivalent amalgam. In relation to the faults seen in the picture, the attainment of a good approximal contact can be difficult because of the softness of the unset composite—it cannot be condensed against a matrix band in the same way as amalgam. Composite does not pass through a carvable phase and, therefore, unless the placement of the matrix is accurate, there will be hard material around the periphery of the restoration. This would be removed by fine polishing diamonds or strips but the approximal area has reduced access and this makes finishing technically difficult.

Material properties
- Polymerisation shrinkage and thermal effects.
  The setting of composite resins is by addition polymerisation, which results in contraction of the material. The forces generated during this contraction will break interfacial bonds between the cavity wall and the material, even if bonding agents are used. Furthermore, the changes in intra-oral temperature during service will result in differential dimensional changes in tooth and material, again causing deterioration in adaptation. The result is an interspace between the cavity wall and the material into which ions in solution and bacteria can pass. This is known as microleakage. The effects may be sensitivity, pulpal irritation, recurrent caries and stained margins.
- Ageing of the resin.
  The dimethacrylates used as the matrix in composite materials are affected by ultraviolet light and UV absorbers are added to the formulation to enhance the colour stability. The polymer absorbs water and over some years may oxidise. A further source of colour instability is the deterioration of the amine used as an initiator in the setting reaction. The effect of all these factors is to cause yellowing of the material, as seen in *Figure 85*. Current photoactivated materials use less amine and are more colour stable than chemically activated materials.

91 (a) They are due to recurrent caries under the mesial amalgam restoration. The light band indicates the outward extension of enamel caries and the dark band the discoloured caries of the dentine.

(b) The caries in this situation is likely to be extensive and may have seriously affected the pulp. A history should be taken to confirm the absence or otherwise of pulpitic symptoms. The extent of the caries needs to be determined by its removal with the gentle use of burs and careful excavation without anaesthesia to establish the integrity of the pulp. If no exposure is found, pulp vitality should be confirmed with a pulp test unless the patient has already indicated sensitivity during cavity preparation. A positive result will indicate that a standard restoration will suffice. If pulpitic symptoms, a pulpal exposure or a negative vitality response exist, pulp treatment will have to precede restoration.

92 (a) The veneer has been made from a castable ceramic (Dicor[15]) stained on the surface to provide the desired colour and aesthetics. The margins have been adjusted with a rotary instrument after fitting. This has removed some of the surface staining, exposing the underlying colourless glass and giving rise to the dark appearance.

(b) Adjustment of bulky contours at the margins of ceramic laminate veneers should not be necessary if sufficient tooth preparation has been undertaken and the standard of technical work is satisfactory. Excess resin at margins can be removed without resorting to instrumentation that damages ceramic. Castable glass ceramics provide excellent marginal fit and there should be no need to adjust them. Lack of preparation space in this case resulted in overbuilt margins with a poor emergence profile.

(c) Most other laminate systems use ceramics in which the colour is dispersed through the body of the material. Adjustment of such materials would not alter the colour significantly unless the underlying tooth was particularly dark.

(d) Repair of this defect would be difficult. Dicor glass can be etched successfully in the mouth, with suitable precautions, using buffered hydrofluoric acid gels or acidulated phosphate fluoride gels. A thin layer of composite resin could then be bonded over the defect to replace the missing stain. A more drastic alternative would be to remove the existing veneer and replace it after making sure all remnants of ceramic and resin had been removed from the enamel surface. This is a difficult procedure and there is a risk that the colour match of the replacement may not be satisfactory.

93 (a) A cervical retention groove is being placed at the gingival margin of the Class V cavity in the upper right central incisor tooth.

(b)

- The acid-etch technique and the application of an intermediary resin for the incisal enamel bond part of the cavity.
- Fresh dentine should be created for bonding, by roughening the dentine with a diamond or cleaning the surface with pumice (water slurry).
- Use of an established dentine bonding system (with a proven record of clinical longevity) according to the manufacturer's instructions.
- The cavity should be restored by placing and curing the composite resin in increments.
- The restoration should be contoured to minimise final finishing.
- Delayed finishing of the cervical dentine margin (> 1/52) of Class V dentine bonded composite restorations is recommended to allow hygroscopic expansion of the resin to compensate for polymerisation contraction.
- Vibration and friction from finishing can damage the composite resin and weaken the composite/dentine bond.

94 (a) *Chemically cured composites* have multiple centres of initiation of polymerisation scattered evenly throughout the setting material. Polymerisation shrinkage will occur evenly throughout the material and will tend to cause generalised contraction towards the centre of the resin mass.

Light-activated resins have the greater concentration of initiation sites at the surface of the resin closest to the light source. As the light is attenuated by its passage through the material, the quality of cure will be reduced. The polymerisation will thus be greatest at the surface of the material and the resin mass will tend to contract towards that surface and hence towards the light source.

(b) A *chemically cured* material will tend to exert even forces upon all areas of the tooth/restoration interface.

A *light-activated* material will contract towards the light source, which will tend to pull the material away from the base/lining material on the cavity floor, leaving a void, or, in Class II restorations, aggravate the problems of maintenance of a good marginal seal.

(c) The detrimental effects of polymerisation contraction include:

- Disruption of the attachment between restoration and tooth with marginal gap formation and microleakage at the interface.

- Distortion of the residual cuspal tissue as a result of maintenance of attachment between tooth and restoration.

In this latter case significant stresses will be set up both with the tooth and within the restorative materials which may have a detrimental effect upon the durability of the restoration.

When any given increment of composite sets there will be an element of plastic flow within the material, dissipating some of the contraction stress. This will be proportionately greater in a small increment of composite than in a large one, and is related to the free surface area of the material.

- An incremental placement technique, designed to maximise the free surface area of each portion to be cured, will help to dissipate the polymerisation stress.
- Equally, attempts should be made to avoid increments extending fully across a cavity to minimise wall-to-wall shrinkage.
- Finally, the increments placed at the gingival floor of a cavity or along the axial walls of the box of a Class II restoration should be cured by transillumination through the tooth so that the materials shrink towards the curing light and, hence the tooth, rather than away from the tooth if an occlusal approach had been used. A light-reflecting wedge may be useful in the proximal areas.

95 (a) Internal bleaching.

(b)
- The tooth is isolated with rubber dam.
- The restoration in the access cavity and root filling are removed to reveal the internal dentine surface.
- The root filling is removed to just below the level of the dento-gingival junction and clear access gained to the area of the pulp horns so that the bleaching agent can reach all internal dentine surfaces.
- A layer of polycarboxylate or glass-ionomer (polyalkenoate) cement is placed over the coronal end of the root filling and allowed to set.
- Phosphoric acid etching solution is applied to the internal surface of the tooth to remove the smear layer and allow better penetration of the bleaching agents into the tubules.
- Bleaching itself is undertaken with 100 vol. (30%) hydrogen peroxide applied on pledgets of cotton wool placed in the access cavity. The application of heat and bright light accelerates the process. The pledgets are replaced at 30 s intervals for approximately 10–15 min. Alternatively, or in addition, the tooth can be sealed with a stiff paste, made by mixing the hydrogen peroxide with sodium perborate, placed on the inner dentine walls. Following this, the access cavity is filled with a pledget of cotton wool and the tooth sealed with polycarboxylate cement.
- At the second visit the tooth is again isolated and the process repeated. If necessary, a third application may be required.
- Once a satisfactory shade has been achieved, the tooth is isolated, again with rubber dam, the dressing removed and any bleaching paste carefully washed out.
- The access cavity is restored with a colour-matched glass-ionomer (polyalkenoate) cement which, if subjected to substantial occlusal stress, can be covered with composite restorative material.

(c) Complications of the technique that may occur include:
- *External cervical resorption.* Placement of a base over the root filling attempts to restrict the bleaching agent to the cavity, preventing its escape along dentinal tubules to the external surface.
- *Seepage of the agents beneath the rubber dam.* A protective layer of vaseline around the neck of the tooth should prevent, or at least limit, such damage from occurring.

- *Insufficient colour change.* Care should be taken to ensure that all the existing restoration has been removed from the tooth so that the bleaching agent can come into direct contact with the discoloured dentine. The expiry date of the solution and its method of storage should both be checked. A lighter shade of restorative material may be attempted.

96
- In some cases simply polishing the amalgam restoration would be sufficient.
- If the restoration is otherwise intact and there is no secondary caries it may be possible to cut back the visible part of the amalgam and face the area with composite, acid etching it to the rim of enamel and using a bonding agent to assist retention to the amalgam.
- If the restoration has other faults it should be replaced. The options are to replace it with a porcelain inlay, a laboratory-made composite inlay, a chairside composite restoration or, if the patient does not object to the appearance of gold, a gold inlay.

What should not be done is to convert this intracoronal restoration to an extracoronal one, i.e. a crown, because this would be much more destructive and there is a large amount of buccal enamel present which has a good appearance.

97 (a) (iii) Air turbine cutting at 300,000 rev/min with water spray coolant. Cutting with a conventional engine above 3000 rev/min would also require water coolant to prevent pulpal damage.
(b) (ii) The earliest microscopic changes in the pulp of a careless cavity preparation is the displacement of odontoblastic nuclei material into dentinal tubules.
(c) (i) Pain associated with changes of temperature indicates pulpal inflammation. The symptoms may resolve if a sedative dressing is placed or they may progress to loss of pulp vitalty and apical periodontitis.

98 (a) Amalgam DO restorations in the upper second premolar and first molar have considerable cervical excess and poor approximal contours.
(b) The faults could have been prevented by tight cervical wedging and burnishing of the matrix band with a ball-ended instrument to give it convexity. A good condensation technique will produce a strong amalgam and will ensure good contours and tight contacts when the matrix is removed.

99 (a) For a single restoration, the main advantage is that the material can be light-cured on its fitting surface whereas with a direct material the light may not penetrate to this depth. This problem with direct materials should be minimised by incremental packing, keeping the increments to a maximum thickness of 2 mm.
   A further advantage of the indirect technique is that the interproximal contour can be optimised. Finally, polymerisation shrinkage takes place on the model and any space is subsequently filled by the cementing composite.
   The disadvantage is that the procedure is extremely time-consuming and in reality there is probably very little to be gained from this indirect chairside technique.
(b) By exposing the inlays to heat and light or heat and pressure it is possible to increase the degree of conversion of the material, i.e the % of C=C which polymerises to crosslink the matrix. For multiple restorations, especially in one quadrant, it is much quicker to take an impression and send it to the laboratory than to spend chairside time contouring each restoration. The contour and contact points of multiple restorations may be improved.
(c) A composite material with small filler particles and a dual system of initiation (light and chemical).

100 (a) This area exhibits white patches which are white spot lesions, indicative of enamel caries, in conjunction with a tooth-coloured restoration.

(b) The brown staining on the labial aspect of the lateral incisor is exogenous stain picked up by a white spot lesion from drinks like tea, coffee and red wine.

(c) The enamel around the filling on the labial aspect of the upper right central incisor is discoloured and this may look unsightly when the patient smiles. If so it will probably necessitate replacement. However, this operative work will not prevent further decay. If this is a new patient it will be important to try to assess whether the lesions are active, in need of preventive treatment, or arrested, requiring monitoring. If in doubt, active caries should be assumed and the lesion treated preventively as well as operatively!

101 For optimal activity of sterilisation procedures, all visible debris should first be removed from the instrument. Adherent cement and other visible contamination should be removed in an ultrasonic cleaning bath; debridement by hand is less efficient, may result in damage to instruments and is potentially hazardous to the operator.

Following gross decontamination, the instrument should be sterilised by heat, either by autoclaving ($134^{\circ}C$ for 4 min) or by incubation in a hot air oven ($180^{\circ}C$ for 30 min).

Cold-sterilisation procedures using disinfectant solutions are less reliable and require long immersion times to be effective. These methods should be reserved for the sterilisation of instruments and equipment which cannot be sterilised by heat.

102 (a) A combination of events may have contributed to the cause of the ulcer:
- The vasoconstrictor in the local anaesthetic will have caused an area of relative tissue ischaemia.
- As the tooth has been restored with composite resin, there may have been careless handling of orthophosphoric acid used in the acid-etching technique. This will have damaged the compromised alveolar mucosa and led to ulceration of the tissue.
- It is also possible that a cotton wool roll 'burn' may have occurred.

(b) Accepting that a mental block rather than an inferior dental block was the most appropriate local anaesthetic, care should have been taken to place the local anaesthetic slowly, attempting to avoid blanching the tissue to any appreciable extent. Use of a carefully applied rubber dam which successfully sealed the gingival margins of the prepared and adjoining teeth would have prevented the acid from affecting the soft tissues and would have obviated the need for cotton wool rolls. Use of acid-etch in a strongly coloured gel form allows more controlled placement and it will be less likely to escape unnoticed onto mucosa. When washed from the margins of a cavity the operator should always check that no etchant remains on the soft tissues.

(c) The local anaesthetic cartridge contains:
- A local anaesthetic drug (or drugs).
- A vasoconstrictor.
- Buffers (to maintain pH).
- Sterile, distilled water.
- NaCl (incorporated to produce an isotonic solution).
- An antiseptic.
- A preservative.

The local anaesthetic is likely to be delivered in one of two forms: 2% Lignocaine (anaesthetic agent) with 1:80,000 adrenaline (vasoconstrictor) or 3% Prilocaine (anaesthetic) with 0.03 iu/ml felypressin (vasoconstrictor).

'Plain' local anaesthetic is available (e.g. 3% Mepivacaine) for use when a vasoconstrictor is contraindicated. The anaesthetic itself exerts a limited vasoconstrictor effect but the action of the drug is of much shorter duration as the bloodstream dissipates the anaesthetic.

103 (a) There has been considerable alveolar resorption in the saddle area, as witnessed by the position of the incisive papilla. In addition there is marked gingival recession associated with the upper left canine. If the preparation was to be extended to the gum margin in this area, difficulty would be experienced by the operator in trying to create a shouldered finishing line on a tapering root surface.

(b)
• The provision of a well-retained metal-based tooth-supported partial denture.
• Implants.
• A precision retained removal anterior bridge.

(c) The only suitable fixed bridge would be a fixed–fixed design. Because of the length of span, a minimum of four abutments would be appropriate, using full-coverage metal–ceramic crowns, limiting the depth of preparation on the labial surface of the upper left canine as previously indicated.

104 Missing or peg-shaped upper lateral incisors are a common developmental anomaly. These teeth may also exhibit malformation of the cingulum area, ranging from deep cingulum pits to dens in dente. The treatment options will depend on the extent of the malformation and the degree to which the patient is disturbed by the abnormal aesthetics.

• Increasing the size of a peg lateral is complicated by the small root, which leads to an unsatisfactory gingival margin where the wider crown or veneer joins it. There may also be insufficient space to accommodate a wider tooth, in which case orthodontics should be considered.
• The orthodontic options are to open the space to allow an increase in width of the restorations, or to extract the peg laterals and close the space, bringing the canines forward. This latter option can make the aesthetics worse if the canines are large despite recontouring the incisal tips.
• Where sufficient space exists and where the malformed laterals are large enough to receive restorations, the choice is between adding acid-etch retained composite tips, providing ceramic veneers and full-coverage ceramic jacket crowns. The composite tip is easy to provide and little tooth reduction is usually necessary. The disadvantage is that the margins or the surface of the material may stain. The veneer provides a good and lasting colour but tooth reduction is necessary and an impression stage with laboratory support is also required. Veneers are vulnerable to chipping where there is an unsatisfactory incisal relationship. The full crown requires the removal of much more tooth, but the result is stronger than the veneer and the fitting stage is much less demanding in terms of shade matching and bonding.

The lateral incisors in *Figure 97* have good enamel and root quality and are slightly short and angled mesially. The treatment provided was to add composite to the distal corners and then to reshape the teeth, removing the mesial corners to correct the angulation.

105 Both operative and prosthetic aspects require consideration.

Design. This covers features of both fixed and removable appliances, inlay cavities and those for plastic restorations.

• Appliances. If fixed, they should be adequately supported and retained on periodontally sound teeth, with appropriate distribution of load (narrowing of occlusal tables and a reduction of cusp slopes) so no detrimental forces hasten bone loss. Embrasures must allow satisfactory interdental cleaning. Removable appliances should also incorporate a load-distribution element and there should be no tilting forces on abutments in order to minimise periodontal breakdown. Teeth used for retention must be braced.
• Wherever feasible, intra- and extracoronal restorations should not encroach upon gingival margins and attention should be paid to the 3 mm rule in partial denture design.

- Food stagnation around the necks of teeth should be avoided and prevented.
- Temporary coverage should reproduce correct occlusal contours to prevent tooth movement or initiate periapical trauma. The margins must be smooth to avoid the accumulation of plaque which would lead to gingival inflammation and hyperplasia or recession.

Preparation

(a) Trauma to gum margins during cavity preparation is unlikely to have long-lasting effects or initiate dental disease. However, deep sub-gingival extensions should be avoided and if caries or a fracture dictates the position of a margin, mucogingival surgery can be considered.
(b)
- There must be complete elimination of peripheral caries.
- Weakened cusps require support to prevent fracture in function.
- Parallelism will be necessary for the retention of extracoronal restorations, especially when used as bridge retainers. This will prevent undiagnosed debonding from leading to the development of recurrent caries.

(c) There must be controlled cavity preparation to prevent pulp damage.

Completion

- Restoration surfaces should be smooth and polished.
- Abnormal contours allow plaque retention and these require modification. This applies to both fixed and removable appliances.
- Fixed appliances must allow interdental cleaning.
- Margins of cast restorations should not be overextended or allow plaque accumulation by being deficient.
- Cervical excess must be removed.
- The occlusion of all restorations should reproduce the normal so that periodontal support is not stressed.
- The presence of marginal ridges and interdental sluices helps to maintain gingival health.

106 (a) The most appropriate means of retaining the restorations in the teeth would be with a dual-cured composite luting resin. The technique involves etching enamel and dentine using a 'total etch' procedure to make the enamel surface mechanically retentive and to remove mineral from the smear layer on the dentine. A hydrophilic dentine bonding resin is applied to enamel and dentine before sealing the surface with a thin layer of unfilled resin. The restoration surfaces are etched in the laboratory with hydrofluoric acid and coated with silane to promote a bond to the luting resin.
(b) The ceramic has a natural translucency similar to enamel and is bonded with resin of similar optical properties and refractive index. It is therefore difficult to detect the lute line because light is transmitted and scattered similarly through tooth, luting resin and restoration.
(c)
- The resin lute is far less resistant to abrasion than the ceramic or tooth and will wear preferentially. This results in slight defects at the restoration margins which, after some considerable time, may become unsupported and chip.
- Another possibility is that the ceramic may wear, producing a rough surface which abrades the opposing tooth. This is dependent on the type of ceramic used and the quality of finish produced at the time of placement.

107 (a) The crown of the tooth could be restored with amalgam, composite resin, glass-ionomer (polyalkenoate) or cermet cement using pins or posts for additional retention. Alternatively, the tooth could be prepared to receive a cast post and core.
(b) Amalgam is generally the core material of choice in the posterior quadrants and in this instance pins or posts would not be required to augment retention as considerable coronal

tooth tissue remains. Retention could be gained from undercuts placed in the pulp chamber walls and from condensing amalgam into the prepared pulp chamber as part of the build-up for the amalgam core. Placement of pins and posts would involve unnecessary effort and the additional risk of possible root perforation.

108 (a) The discoloration is grey–brown and appears to have a chronological basis. The most likely cause is ingestion of tetracycline as a child. The patient or her parents should be questioned about long-standing childhood illnesses, especially chest infections.
(b) The discoloration is intrinsic within the dentine and enamel. The management strategies should be designed to disguise the dentine by modifying or covering the enamel surface. Options include:
- *Vital bleaching*, using either acid etching and heat/light-activated hydrogen peroxide at the chairside, or peroxide/amine home bleaching kits in a custom tray. The method of action is unsure, although there may be some modification of the optical properties of the enamel to help mask the underlying dentine.
- *Veneers*, using either direct-placement composite resin restorations or laboratory-made composite resin or porcelain veneers. The latter are attached to the tooth surface using a composite resin luting agent after acid etching the enamel.
- *Crowns*, either as minimal-preparation veneer crowns or in the form of conventional porcelain or porcelain fused to metal restorations.
(c) Management at this age should be based upon minimal tooth destruction. The dental pulp is still large and may interfere with full-crown preparation. The gingival contour of teeth is not stable, so further apical migration might be expected, exposing underlying tooth tissue. This will be different in colour to any restoration, necessitating their relatively early replacement.

The first approach would probably be to attempt vital bleaching, using a peroxide/amine system. If only partially successful, this could be followed by the placement of a veneer. As the severity of the discoloration will have been reduced, there will be less requirement of the veneer to provide a masking effect. In these circumstances the optical properties of the veneering material could be chosen to give better aesthetics. The material of choice at this age would probably be a microfine composite resin. A porcelain veneer could then be used to replace such restorations in the patient's early 20s once the gingival contour becomes more stable.

109 (a) Initial treatment would, in this case, involve the removal of the carious and stained dentine and the placement of an amalgam core. The use of glass-ionomer (polyalkenoate) cement would not be ideal as a substantial amount of tooth tissue is missing. A composite core, while being strong enough, would be less retentive than amalgam because of the shrinkage on setting which will occur. Marginal percolation is also a problem with this type of core material, again because of polymerisation contraction.
(b) The absence of a substantial portion of both lingual cusps indicates that some type of auxiliary retention will be required. Preferably this should be achieved by the use of pins. The preferred type are those which self-shear. Care must be taken to ensure that the pins are supported by an adequate amount of dentine and that they do not further weaken the tooth structure. Their angulation must be carefully controlled to avoid perforation either of the pulp chamber or into the periodontal ligament space.
(c) Long-term treatment of the tooth should include the provision of some form of crown to protect the remaining tooth substance. In this case a full gold veneer crown would provide a durable and stable structure with minimal reduction of tooth tissue. This is particularly important as the removal of substantial buccal tooth tissue could result in the displacement of the core.

110 (a)
- In this case the resin-bonded bridge has simply been cemented in position with no prior preparation of the teeth. Hence, no occlusal rest has been incorporated into the framework on the mesial surface of the upper premolar.
- Retainer wings for resin-bonded bridges should, ideally, achieve 180° 'wrap around' in order to provide maximum surface area of enamel for bonding. Here there is inadequate extension of the wing distally on the premolar and cervically and mesially on the central incisor.
- Careful consideration of occlusal contacts in centric and excursive movements of the mandible should be checked prior to cementation of any bridgework. In the bridge illustrated in *Figure 102* gross adjustment of the mesial retainer wing suggests this may not have been done.

(b) Tooth preparation should provide:
- Adequate occlusal clearance. In the case of an anterior bridge the minimum thickness of the metal retainer wing should be 0.5 mm.
- A positive seat for the framework created by the incorporation of cingulum and occlusal rests.
- A supra-gingival chamfer finishing margin to allow a smooth transition between the framework and tooth. In cases where abutment teeth are bulbous this may not be possible without cutting into dentine; hence a knife-edge margin would be acceptable.
- Guide planes and approximal grooves to provide a single path of insertion.

(c) The key features to be checked at try-in are:
- Marginal fit.
- Occlusion in all excursions of the mandible.
- Pontic relationship to the edentulous ridge.
- Aesthetics.

111 The gingival margin of these restorations lies on dentine. What has almost certainly happened is that light-cured composite was placed into shallow cavities, similar to those in the lower jaw, and that, although dentine bonding agent may have been used, the polymerisation contraction of the composite in an axial direction has pulled the composite away from the neck of the cavity. The micro-mechanical bond to the etched enamel at the incisal end of the cavity develops more rapidly than the physico-chemical bond, via dentine bonding agent to the dentine. The solution is either to use a glass-ionomer (polyalkenoate) base attached to the dentine and then a thin veneer of composite over the surface, or to apply the composite incrementally from the neck down, curing small increments at a time and finishing with the layer attached to enamel.

112 (a) The elastomeric impression materials available can be classified as:
- Addition-cured silicones (polyvinylsiloxanes).
- Polyethers.
- Condensation-cured silicones.
- Polysulphides.

(b) *Addition-cured silicones* are the most accurate and dimensionally stable of all the elastomers. The materials have good powers of elastic recovery and can be stored for long periods without loss of accuracy. They are capable of good reproduction of surface detail and have a moderate tear strength. Addition-cured silicones are available in a range of consistencies which are easy to use and have a short–medium working time.

Polyethers have very good dimensional stability if stored dry, excellent reproduction of surface detail and a moderate–low tear strength. Elasticity develops rapidly from the time of mixing and it is therefore important that the impression is seated as soon as possible and held undisturbed until set to avoid the introduction of stresses into the material which will lead to its distortion. The material, once set, is relatively hard and difficulty may be experienced in its removal from the mouth, especially if there are areas of pronounced undercut. This hardness may also create difficulty in model construction as thin unsupported cusp preparations may fracture when attempts are made to remove the dies from the impression. Polyethers are easy to use although patients may complain of their bitter taste. They have a short–medium working time.

Condensation-cured silicones are very accurate if the model is poured immediately but are dimensionally unstable on storage because they shrink due to the evaporation of ethanol, a by-product of the polymerisation process. They record surface detail well and have excellent elastic properties but a low tear strength. They are less expensive than addition-cured silicones and polyethers.

Polysulphide impression materials have good flow properties and high flexibility and tear strength. They are capable of recording fine surface detail in the presence of moisture because they are slightly hydrophilic. The materials are sufficiently stable if cast within 30 min but because the setting reaction produces water they shrink with time due to its evaporation. They have a long working time and a relatively long polymerisation time which may add to patient discomfort. Their resistance to deformation is low and they have a bad taste and odour. Generally, their use demands the construction of a special tray in order to control polymerisation shrinkage by the use of a uniform thickness of impression material.

113 (a) The patient will have been given chlorhexidine mouthwash to prevent post-operative wound infection. This has resulted in chlorhexidine staining of the teeth and composite restorations.
(b) Glycoprotein pellicles form on all surfaces in the mouth. These are rapidly colonised by bacteria, resulting in the formation of plaque, which increases in thickness as a network of glycoprotein, bacteria and associated polysaccharides. However, if the number of bacteria is reduced by the presence of chlorhexidine, the glycoprotein pellicle may increase in thickness. This thickened pellicle becomes stained as a result of interaction with the diet and chlorhexidine. The exact staining mechanism is not fully understood: some researchers believe it to be the passive absorption of dietary stain into the pellicle, while others believe that chlorhexidine chemically reacts with the pellicle enabling it to bind ions such as sulphur.
(c) None at all. In this case the stained pellicle will be worn away as soon as the chlorhexidine therapy has been completed. However, if the staining occurs in marginal gaps it can be extremely difficult to remove.
(d) Some patients with chronic periodontal disease are encouraged to use this mouthwash on a regular basis. This will lead to staining of the composite restorations, which may be an aesthetic problem if they involve visible surfaces at the front of the mouth.

114 (a) Sjögren's syndrome is an autoimmune connective tissue disorder. Principally it affects the salivary and lachrymal glands which become damaged by lymphatic infiltrates and therefore produce less secretion: 15–30% of patients with rheumatoid arthritis also have Sjögren's syndrome.
(b) The dry mouth of Sjögren's syndrome makes these patients particularly susceptible to dental caries. *Figure 105* shows lesions developing in the dentine on the incisal aspects of the lower incisors.
(c) The lesion in the lower right central incisor would be managed operatively as well as preventively if the dentine was soft to probing. Hard lesions are either arrested or may be arrested by improved cleaning, taking care with the diet and with the sensible use of fluoride.

- The impression should be rinsed in tap water to remove blood and secretions, and then placed in a sealed container marked with a biohazard warning for transport to the laboratory.
- On arrival at the laboratory the impression should be removed from its container with a gloved hand and placed in a fresh aqueous solution of gluteraldehyde for 3 h or overnight.
- At the end of this period the impression may be removed, again by a gloved hand, rinsed in water and cast in the usual manner.

116 (a) Electrosurgery.

(b) *Indications:*

- For removal of hyperplastic gingival tissue (as pictured) where it has proliferated into cavities or over crown preparations.
- It can be used in place of a gingival retraction cord to facilitate an impression of a deep sub-gingival fracture.
- Some operators use the technique routinely in place of gingival retraction where substantial attached gingiva is present.
- It may also be used for crown-lengthening procedures prior to the provision of crowns.

Contraindications:

- As it may interfere with function, use on or in the vicinity of people wearing cardiac pacemakers is a major contraindication.
- Use should be avoided with patients who are being treated with nitrous oxide/oxygen analgesia (RA) to prevent any sparks which arise leading to a flash fire in the oxygen-rich environment.
- Where attached gingival tissue is thin, or where an underlying dehiscence is suspected (e.g. buccally on upper canines) gingival recession may be marked following use of this technique and should be considered before electrosurgery is contemplated.

117 (a) The patient is suffering from chronic marginal gingivitis, probably caused by poor crown margins. This may result from either the cement lute being dissolved, thus allowing plaque to accumulate in the space, or from positive edges. These may directly traumatise the gingivae or again harbour plaque because of cleansing difficulties.

(b) In order for the condition to improve it will be necessary to remove the predisposing factors and improve the oral hygiene. If the crown margins can be modified at the chairside this may be sufficient to allow adequate cleaning. It may, however, be necessary to remove them and arrange for some good fitting acrylic temporary crowns to be constructed in the laboratory. These must be checked for accuracy of fit and, following cementation, the patient instructed in appropriate cleaning methods.

Once the tissue inflammation has resolved, the preparations should be modified if necessary and accurate impressions sent to the laboratory for new permanent crowns to be made.

If no improvement in gingival contour is achieved, thought may have to be given to the use of surgery.

Prior to cementing the new crowns, they must again be carefully inspected to ensure that none of the original errors have been perpetuated or new ones incorporated.

118 (a) This syndrome is associated with a crack in the enamel extending to the ADJ or more usually into the dentine itself, which allows flexing of the dentine—and thus stimulation of pulpal nerves—and results in a painful 'hyperaemic'-type response.

(b) The tooth concerned may be difficult to identify. Most teeth exhibit superficial cracks in the enamel and it is often impossible to distinguish between these and the offending deep crack. The patient may be convinced that a particular tooth is to blame but the symptoms of pulpal hyperaemia are notoriously unreliable. It may be possible to identify the offending tooth by getting the patient to bite tooth-to-tooth on something hard, like the handle of a dental instrument, or by applying a small pledget of cotton wool and ethyl chloride, to see if either can induce a matching sensation to that of which the patient complains. Failing this it will be necessary to select the most likely tooth to have fractured in the quadrant under investigation—such as the most heavily filled one with the steepest cusps—and remove the restoration to allow inspection of the dentine in the cavity floor. The crack may then be obvious or it may be a mere hairline, in which case it can often be revealed by the application of a disclosing solution. If nothing is revealed it will be necessary to move to the next likely tooth.

119 (a) If the cervical margin extends below the cemento-enamel junction, then the possibility of secondary caries is increased. The glass-ionomer (polyalkenoate) leaches fluoride ions, reducing the solubility of the root dentine.
(b) When glass-ionomers were externalised interproximally under composite restorations, the material dissolved away over a number years leaving a gap at the cervical margin (Welbury and Murray, 1990). This effect has been attributed to the low pH that can occur interproximally as a result of plaque metabolism. In this acid environment the glass-ionomer dissolves away.
(c) The patient was 78 years old and had developed quite severe root caries interproximally. In this case it was felt that the ability of the material to prevent secondary caries outweighed the possibility of its dissolution.
(d) In this case a Type II reinforced material; but under a composite, a Type II aesthetic glass-ionomer cement.

120 (a) The surface preparation is macro-mechanical, sometimes described as Virginia Salt Loss or Crystal Bond[16] bridge.
(b) The undercuts are created by coating the die with salt crystals or acrylic beads which become incorporated into the wax pattern. The former are dissolved in water before investing and casting or, in the case of the acrylic, are burnt out in the furnace; both allow the formation of a re-entrant surface.
(c) *Advantages*
• No special laboratory equipment is required.
• The bonding resin is fully protected by the metal retainer.
• Debonded retainers can easily be cleaned and rebonded.
Disadvantages
• Retainers must be greater than 0.6 mm in thickness to make room for the macroscopic pores.
• Retention stops short of the retainer margins by 0.5–1 mm (*Figure 110*).
• Removal of the pattern to dissolve the salt which creates the undercuts may cause distortion and reduce the accuracy of fit.
• Air trapped in the fitting surface may inhibit the set of some chemically adhesive resins.
(d) Other methods of bonding to metal include:
• Perforated metal wings (Rochette).
• Metal mesh.
• Gel or electrolytically etched non-precious alloy (Maryland).
• Alumina grit-blasted non-precious alloy and chemical adhesives.
• Tin-plated precious metal alloys.
• Silane-coated alloys.

121 (a) *Advantages*:
- The creation of a definite finishing line during preparation identifies the limits of the enamel requiring etching.
- Tooth preparation before veneering allows a restoration to be made with less risk of over-contour. In addition to providing a better appearance, this simplifies plaque control for the patient.
- The technician is provided with a cast upon which the area to be covered by the veneer and the margins may be readily identified.
- Incisal reduction and the production of a cervical finishing line aid the clinician with the correct seating of the veneer at try-in and during cementation.
- Removal of some enamel during tooth preparation may enhance bonding via the acid-etch technique by the removal of an aprismatic or less readily etched surface enamel. This may also simplify the masking of discoloured areas by reducing the intensity or extent of any discoloured areas.

Disadvantages:
- Tooth preparation makes the procedure irreversible.
- There is risk of exposing dentine, especially cervically. As well as causing sensitivity and possible pulpal irritation there is a significant risk of marginal microleakage, leading to marginal discoloration and secondary caries.

(b)
- *Appearance*: the veneer should be tried in wet with either a drop of water or glycerine to obtain a reliable estimate of the possible post-cementation appearance with a clear bonding cement.
- *Marginal fit/extension*: multiple veneers should be tried in separately, then together.
- *Occlusal relationships*: these should be checked in all functional occlusal excursions.

(c)
- The veneer fit surface should be cleaned to remove any saliva contamination or try-in composite.
- If the fit surface has not previously been treated with silane and protected with light-cured unfilled resin this should be done at this stage.
- The enamel surface should be cleaned with pumice and water or an oil-free fluoride prophylaxis paste.
- While protecting adjacent teeth with matrix strips, the enamel is acid-etched.
- The etched surface is washed and dried and a layer of unfilled bond resin is applied and blow thinned.
- An appropriate shade of light-cured composite is applied to the fit surface of the veneer which is 'puddled' into place on the tooth surface.
- Gross excess of composite should be removed and light-curing completed.
- Remaining excess composite is removed with finishing diamond burs, discs, strips, etc., and the margins finally polished.
- The patient should be reviewed after approximately 1 week.

122 (a) Dental caries superimposed upon wear is unusual. The wear process often involves softening of the tooth surface by some external source and its subsequent removal by direct contact, through the action of a food bolus or with a toothbrush and dentifrice. Caries is fundamentally a process that commences with softening of the surface enamel or dentine. If there is an ongoing wear problem, such lesions would be worn away rather than develop, as in this case. Consequently, this is a reflection of a change in the oral environment, where a previously destructive domain has altered to a cariogenic one.

The pattern of tooth wear, confined to the buccal surfaces of teeth, is compatible with either a dietary habit, exposure to an industrial acidic atmosphere or to an abrasive assault through overly vigorous oral hygiene, possibly with an abrasive dentifrice or, once again, to an industrial cause.

The caries is likely to be dietary in origin, although alterations in salivary function should not be excluded.

(b) Careful questioning concerning diet, oral hygiene methodology and occupation may give a clue to the wear problem. Care must be taken to ask the patient about past experiences rather than current habits, as the problem has apparently stopped.

Dietary and medical history in association with a 3-day diet history may help to clarify the current caries problem.

Once the aetiology of the condition is established, appropriate preventive advice can be given and a treatment plan formulated. It would be inappropriate to proceed with any form of extensive reconstruction if there was an ongoing acidic challenge within the mouth, either from dietary, medical or environmental influences.

(c) The treatment options must first include control of the existing caries with appropriate restorations and preventive advice. The materials chosen for the restorations should be compatible with the longer-term treatment goals for the patient; that is, if a tooth is destined to have a full coronal restoration, an appropriate material for a core should be used rather than one which may produce a better short-term aesthetic result but would then need to be replaced prior to crown preparation.

The tissue loss is sufficiently severe on the upper anterior teeth to warrant full coronal restorations; indeed much of the buccal tissue reduction has already been achieved by the patient! The premolar teeth and the lower anteriors could be managed either by a veneering technique, using composite resin or porcelain, or by full coronal restorations. Obviously, the former is less destructive of residual tooth tissue.

123 (a) For a patient of this age the most appropriate replacement for the missing teeth would be by means of resin-retained bridges.

(b) The movement of canines is often appropriate in these clinical circumstances because it permits space to be created or concentrated where it can be most usefully employed to allow aesthetically sized pontics to be constructed. Their mesial movement, however, may present difficulties, especially if no coronal tooth reduction is anticipated; e.g. where the spaces will be restored by means of a removable partial denture or, as in this case, resin-retained bridges. Here their shape will have to be modified considerably, both in length and breadth, to produce teeth which have the appearance of upper lateral incisors. It would probably have been better to move the canines distally, thus recreating the missing lateral spaces which could then be restored with the resin-retained bridges. This option would eliminate the need to modify the natural tooth contours.

(c) It is essential, in cases of this type, that careful treatment planning is undertaken at the initial stages so that the teeth are moved to a position of maximum advantage. Careful planning is especially important where there is to be collaborative treatment provided by more than one operator. The conservative treatment should be provided once the canines are in a stable upright position, allowing aesthetic pontics to be placed to fill the created spaces.

124 (a) Alloys that can be used in the construction of metal–ceramic crowns include:
- *High gold*: gold (80–90%), platinum and/or palladium, plus small amounts of silver, tin, iron and indium.
- *Gold/palladium*: gold (50%), palladium (30%), tin and indium (10%), and silver.
- *Palladium/silver*: palladium (60%), silver (30%), tin and indium (10%).
- *High palladium alloys*: palladium (> 80%), tin (10–12%).
- *Base metal alloys*: e.g. nickel–chromium systems.

(b) To make the substructure, a wax pattern is prepared, invested using a phosphate-bonded investment and cast. The casting is sandblasted to remove the investment and thoroughly cleaned. Accuracy of fit is verified on the model at this stage. The casting is then degassed in the furnace and, after cooling, a thin opaque slurry is painted onto the substructure and fired at the specific temperature for the alloy concerned. All porcelain firing cycles are carried out under vacuum except the final glaze. A second opaque coating is applied and fired to complete the masking of the substructure. Dentine and enamel shades of porcelain are next applied and contoured following which they are fired. A second firing is normally required for final adjustment of shape and the procedure is completed with the final glaze. The precise temperatures, timings and pressures will be dependent on the specific bonding alloys and porcelains selected.

(c) There are three important components of the metal–ceramic bond:

- *Mechanical*. Surface tension provides intimate contact of the porcelain with the micro-surface irregularities of the metal.
- *Chemical*. The metal oxide film produces a chemical bond with the porcelain.
- *Compressive shrinkage* of the porcelain is resisted by the metal and compressive forces set up in the porcelain.

125 (a) A stainless steel post and composite core is a one-visit procedure and avoids the need for a temporary post crown. It also avoids the contamination of the post hole with temporary cement, which is one of the reasons that some permanent posts and cores become decemented. The strength of a post and core system is limited by its weakest link. If the post is wrought stainless steel, this is usually more reliable and stronger than a cast post which may contain porosity. If the post is long enough to come through to the tip of the core, then it is equally strong throughout its length and adding a metal core would not improve its strength. The composite core, if well retained all round the post, is sufficiently strong.

A disadvantage of the technique is that the post and core must be in a straight line, thus preventing any dramatic alteration in crown position should this be indicated.

(b)
- The 1| preparation has a mesial restoration still present, which is probably a composite that was retained by the enamel. Its retention is therefore now suspect. In addition, there is staining within the dentine beneath the restoration and it would be better to remove this restoration and repair the area with glass-ionomer (polyalkenoate) cement.
- The |1 crown preparation has lost a restoration mesially and this has produced an undercut. It would be better to restore this with glass-ionomer (polyalkenoate) cement now rather than take the impression and block out the area on the die. If this is done, then when the permanent crown is cemented the cavity becomes filled with the luting cement which is likely to be more irritant to the pulp than a glass-ionomer restoration.
- The |2 preparation is undercut between the palatal gingival surface and the depression in the labial surface. This should again be blocked out or the labial surface further reduced. In addition, this preparation has too sharp an angle between the incisal and palatal surfaces, which should, therefore, be modified.

Good features of all four preparations are that the labial shoulders are sufficiently wide for metal–ceramic crowns and that they have been well contoured in line with the gingival margin. This is acceptable when the lip line is such that the margins would show; otherwise, it is preferable to leave the margins supra-gingival.

126
- The caries experience of the patient should be taken into account. If there has been relatively little caries in the mouth and the patient has good oral hygiene and diet and the lesion is small, the lesion should be observed rather than restored. Alternatively, with a patient who has a high caries incidence and for whom preventive measures have not been

successful, then even small lesions should probably be restored. The age of the patient should also be taken into account and if possible the appearance of the tooth on previous radiographs should be compared with the current view.

• The radiographic appearance of the lesion should be assessed for depth. If the lesion is entirely within the enamel and appears not to penetrate to the enamel–dentine junction, preventive measures should be applied and the tooth kept under radiographic review. However, if the radiograph shows that the lesion makes contact with dentine, there is almost certainly irreversible caries within the dentine. Certainly, if the radiolucency is visible within dentine, the tooth must be restored.

127 (a) The lower incisors have mild incisal edge loss but the lower canine has marked loss of enamel with the coronal dentine exposed. The shape of this surface loss matches exactly the contour of the ceramic crown on the upper canine.
(b) The general surface loss is probably the result of parafunction; i.e. tooth-to-tooth grinding with the mouth empty. The effect on the lower canine has been accelerated by the rough surface of the ceramic crown. The crown was probably adjusted at the fitting stage by grinding and then not reglazed. This left a surface which is capable of rapid abrasion of opposing enamel. Poorly finished composite resins may also cause this. The surface of a properly glazed ceramic, while harder than enamel, does not cause abrasion. After clinical adjustments therefore, all ceramic restorations should be reglazed or, if this is not possible, 'polished' with a diamond paste. This has the effect of smoothing the surface but does not impart the protective 'skin' created by glazing.

128 (a) Because of the root fracture.
(b) The root has been considerably weakened by the excessively wide post hole for such a slender tooth. The likelihood of fracture may have been aggravated by interference between the crown and the opposing teeth.
(c) The diameter of the post hole should, if at all possible, have been kept much narrower. This might, however, preclude the use of a cast post as it would be prone to distort if too thin. A wrought or prefabricated post would be stronger and the addition of a bevelled diaphragm would support the root by its 'ferrule' effect and thus resist fracture. Careful assessment and recording of the occlusion would ensure that undue force was not applied by occlusal interference.

129 (a) This is dark brown dentine but there is no obvious cavitation. This is root caries.
(b) Active lesions are soft or leathery, whereas arrested lesions are hard. A probe or excavator should be used gently to determine the consistency of the lesion.
(c) A principal aim of operative treatment is to aid plaque control. Thus, a cavity that was difficult to clean would benefit from a restoration. In addition, a deep, soft lesion would be restored to protect the pulp. Sometimes these lesions show when the patient smiles and a wish to improve appearance might be another reason for operative intervention.

130
• Following glove removal, place the affected hand under running water and allow it to bleed. Bleeding should not be encouraged by sucking.
• Gently wash the wound with detergent.
• Record the incident in the case notes and complete any accident documentation.
• Review the case notes regarding the likely HIV/HBV status of the patient.
• Seek expert medical advice (e.g. General Medical Practitioner, Occupational Health Department, local Haematology Department) regarding the need for further action, including active/passive HBV immunisation, HIV testing/counselling of practitioner or patient.

131 (a) The patient should be questioned regarding their diet, checking especially for an excessive intake of acidic foods or drinks. It is worth asking if anything in particular exacerbates the sensitivity, as this may identify the causative agent. If no abnormal intake is found, discussions with the patient should be directed towards trying to identify if there is any gastric source of acid. This may present as heartburn but, alternatively, may be a sign of bulimia nervosa and the source of the acid not readily disclosed.

(b) If the source of the acid attack can be identified, its role in the tooth surface loss and sensitivity should be explained to the patient. The acid challenge to the tooth can then be reduced. Treatment of the tooth will involve placing a posterior composite resin restoration using a dentine bonding system to cover the exposed, sensitive dentine. Any cavity preparation required should be kept to a minimum.

132 (a) Non-vital teeth can be used:
- As bridge or partial denture abutments.
- For overdenture abutments with or without the addition of precision attachments, often in the form of studs soldered to a cast-gold root cap.
- As a substructure for a post/core restoration.
- If tooth tissue has been lost or there is a danger that remaining tissue may fracture in function the remaining tooth can be restored with a pin- or screw-retained core and the tooth protected by means of a cast restoration.

(b) Aspects that should be considered include:
- Endodontic/periapical status. If canals are unfilled or inadequately obturated, the canal morphology should be assessed.
- Position of the tooth in the arch.
- Integrity of the arch—presence of partial dentures or their needs.
- Hygiene and periodontal status, including the bone support, both general and local.
- Motivation of the patient.
- Age of the patient.
- Restorability of the tooth /root. This should include an assessment of the strength of the remaining tooth substance and consideration of the retention of the final restoration.
- Aesthetics.

(c) Other information that will be necessary will be that gained from:
- A radiographic examination. Certainly a periapical view will be necessary, with the possibility of an overall assessment by means of a dental panoramic tomogram.
- Study models which, if the complexity of the case demands, should be mounted on an articulator so that a full assessment of the occlusion can be undertaken.

133 (a) The metal subframes have been constructed to provide palatal centric stops, rather than using a collar of metal with most of the palatal aspects in ceramic. The metal extends to the incisal third of the crowns.

(b) Metal is easier to adjust clinically when fitting the crowns because it can be repolished using clinical instruments such as impregnated rubber polishing wheels. This is in contrast to ceramic, which requires reglazing or, at the very least, 'polishing' after adjustment with diamond paste. The metal has been extended to the incisal third so that the incisal guidance can be equilibrated easily as well. It is not possible to provide more metal guidance because this would weaken the incisal edge ceramic and decrease the incisal translucency.

134 (a) Some ferric sulphate, used to control bleeding, has remained on the preparation surface and has become reduced to complexes of ferric sulphide, which are black. This discoloration is visible through the ceramic crowns because they have no opaque core, unlike conventional porcelain jacket or porcelain fused to metal crowns. Contamination of the root surface is not noticeable at the time of bonding as the ferric sulphate solution is pale yellow and matches the tooth colour.

(b) The black deposits were found to have a significant thickness when the crowns were removed, indicating a failure of the bond in the area. If crown margins are not fully bonded, sensitivity may be experienced, with the possibility of early mechanical failure because tensile stresses, concentrated at the margin, will not be transferred to the preparation via the resin bond.

(c) The problem may be avoided by blasting the tooth with water and air while delivering the ferric sulphate solution to the gingival crevice with a syringe and special infuser tip.

Thorough mechanical cleaning of the preparation surface must be undertaken before fitting temporary restorations. It is preferable to avoid the use of ferric sulphate at the bonding stage because the tooth surface will become contaminated and cannot be cleaned without some risk of soft-tissue damage and subsequent bleeding. When bonding inlays and onlays, rubber dam will isolate the teeth perfectly. Correct contouring of temporary restorations, careful adaptation of their margins and good oral hygiene, combined with minimal delay in constructing the crowns, will ensure healthy gingival tissues at the bonding stage.

135 (a) *Indications:*
- Well-motivated patient requesting tooth-coloured restorations.
- Good plaque control and periodontal condition.
- Low caries rate.
- Adequate tooth structure for bonding.
- If the restoration is to be a replacement, the outline form of the previous preparation should be free of undercuts or conservatively modifiable.
- All restoration margins should lie on enamel.

Contraindications:
- Previous deep sub-gingival restorations or caries.
- Evidence of bruxism or excessive tooth wear.

(b)
- Occlusal reduction sufficient for > 2 mm material.
- Taper greater than the 3–5° required for gold inlays. Tooth-coloured inlay materials are weak prior to cementation and may, therefore, fracture at try-in.
- Non-undercut cavities with rounded internal line and point angles.
- Butt joint occlusal and cervical cavity margins.
- Buccal/lingual box walls may be bevelled.
- All cavity margins in enamel.
- All exposed dentine cavity surfaces protected with glass-ionomer cement.

(c) *Cast gold onlay.*
- Less tapered preparation.
- Less occlusal reduction (only 0.5-1.0 mm for gold coverage on the non-functional cusps).
- All cavity margins bevelled.

Amalgam will require:
- Butt joint margins.
- 2–3 mm buccal cusp reduction.
- The provision of undercuts or pin placement for retention.

136 (a) The restorations are likely to have failed because of inadequate preparation of the dentine surface, surface contamination during placement of the cement or possibly through flexure of the tooth in function, disrupting the bond between cement and tooth.

(b) Cervical wear lesions of the type shown in an older patient will have an eburnated layer of dentine on the surface of the defect. It has been suggested that bonding to such a dentine layer is poor, but is improved by conditioning the dentine with a surface active agent, e.g. dodicin, or with a mild acid, e.g. poly(acrylic) acid/tannic acid. Poly(acrylic) acid is now provided by most manufacturers of these cements as a dentine surface treatment. An alternative approach would be to instrument the dentine surface gently with a bur in a slow handpiece.

Contamination of a dentine surface with saliva after cavity preparation but prior to placement of the cement will have a marked effect upon the bond between cement and tooth, as the layer of precipitated salivary proteins on the dentine surface will act as a barrier to the necessary chemical interactions at that interface. Such salivary proteins can be removed using the dentine conditioner poly(acrylic) acid with return of bond strengths to their normal values.

(c) Glass-ionomer (polyalkenoate) cements:
• Adhere to mineralised tooth tissue.
• Are tooth coloured, with aesthetics similar to dentine.
• Have the potential to inhibit the development of recurrent caries at their margins as a result of fluoride release from the surface of the set cement.
• In addition, they have the potential to absorb fluoride when local ionic concentrations are high and then release the fluoride slowly when the environmental concentration decreases, thus acting as a fluoride sponge.

(d) Glass-ionomer cements have a low pH when freshly mixed (pH 2) as a result of the polyacid. The mineral component of enamel and dentine is dissolved at this pH, which will partially neutralise the acidity within the cement, resulting in a mineral soup at the cement–tooth interface, comprising Ca^{2+} and PO_4^{2-} ions from the tooth mineral and Ca^{2+}, Al^{3+} and polyacid ions from the cement. The setting reaction of the cement further raises the pH of the setting cement which reaches a critical level at which the mineral soup undergoes a precipitation reaction. During this precipitation, carboxylate groups from the polyacid become incorporated in the mineral on the tooth surface, displacing PO_4^{2-} ions into the cement, and thus binding the cement to the tooth surface.

137 (a) The enamel shows evidence of white opaque areas (mottled enamel) suggestive of enamel hypoplasia due to fluoride. Although there is little mottling of any significance below 0.9–1.0 ppm of fluoride in the water, it becomes progressively evident above this level. While fluoride has been shown to protect teeth against dental caries by reducing the solubility of enamel and promoting its remineralisation after the carious attack, once the lesion has entered into dentine, particularly via a small occlusal fissure, it will progress at a normal rate. In view of the apparent low susceptibility to caries, no previous bitewing radiographs had been taken of this patient, allowing the lesion to progress to this size before detection.

(b) In this case no symptoms had been experienced by the patient and the tooth gave a normal response to vitality tests. After securing anaesthesia of the tooth and isolation with rubber dam, the fissure should be entered and enlarged until the full extent of the lesion can be visualised. Caries should then be removed either with a large round bur, slowly rotating, or with a sharp large excavator, clearing the periphery of the lesion before progressing towards the pulpal floor. Where it is felt that to continue removal of softened dentine would result in exposure of the pulp, excavation should stop and a setting calcium hydroxide cement placed on the pulpal floor. A suitable structural base and restorative material is chosen according to the final size of the cavity.

(c) The patient should be advised of the need for regular dental examinations to prevent similar occurrences from, potentially, going undetected.

138 (a)
- Ideally, composite resin should be used only to restore minimal cavities in posterior teeth. Its use should be restricted to those instances where it will not be subjected to excessive occlusal forces and where, when teeth are in occlusion, there is cusp-to-cusp contact and not cusp to restoration.
- The material is ideal for core techniques where missing tooth substance is replaced prior to preparation for a full or partial crown.
- It is possible to consider the use of the material where aesthetics is an important consideration, such as mesial restorations in the upper first premolar teeth.
- Where excessive tissue removal would be necessary to provide adequate mechanical retention for amalgam.
- Its use may be considered of value where there is excessive internal weakening of the tooth so that the adhesive nature of the material can provide cross-linkage, thus preventing fracture of the tooth.

(b)
- Occlusal surfaces should not be bevelled in an attempt to increase retention as these thin margins will wear in function and precipitate early failure of the restoration.
- The use of Type III glass-ionomer (polyalkenoate) as a base or a dentine bonding agent will aid retention of the final restoration if the floor of the cavity is in dentine.
- Moisture control is necessary in order to achieve effective retention.
- Incremental curing will ensure that the depth of the restoration is completely cured and reduce cuspal flexure.
- The use of prismatic wedges and clear matrix bands will also help guarantee adequate curing of the composite.
- In order to assist contact point formation when composite is used to restore Class II lesions the tooth should be pre-wedged.

139 (a) This is known as the 'soft-tissue' or 'gum-work' technique and the model consists of conventional die stone (α-hemihydrate) and a resilient material which reproduces the gingival contour. Proprietary silicone rubber is available to construct the gingival component but an alternative and more robust 'soft tissue' can be made by mixing self-curing soft denture relining material with conventional polymethylmethacrylate polymer in a ratio of 2:1 prior to mixing with monomer.
(b) The construction of the crowns will be aided as the technician will be able to visualise the relationship of the crown margin to the gingival sulcus. Furthermore, during build-up of the porcelain, the effect of producing a greater or lesser cervical bulbosity will be seen; i.e. the emergence profile will be made to harmonise with the surrounding soft tissue. The technique is also helpful when a metal cervical collar is planned for the crown, or a diaphragm is indicated but the patient is reluctant to show cervical gold.

140 (a) (ii) A Black's Class II cavity involves proximal surfaces of posterior (molars and premolars) teeth. The occlusal surface is included in the outline only as a means of gaining access to the lesion. All the other three descriptions are therefore incorrect.
(b) (i)–(v) inclusive. All these aspects have an important role to play in the maintenance of periodontal health. A correct occlusal contour ensures that the periapical tissues are not traumatised while the remaining features prevent either plaque retention or more direct trauma to the gingival tissues.
(c) (iii) Pulpal caries should be dealt with as the final stage of cavity preparation with the exception, perhaps, of finishing the cavity margins. This allows the cavity outline to be determined and the amelo–dentinal junction to be rendered caries-free and unsupported enamel removed. Whether all pulpal caries is removed or stained but hard tissue retained is

dependent on clinical judgement. A indirect pulp-capping procedure may also be advisable in an attempt to encourage remineralisation and maintain pulp vitality.

141 (a) The following design options should be considered:
- A simple cantilever bridge from the canine or the canine and first premolar.
- A fixed–fixed bridge between canine and central incisor.
- A spring cantilever bridge from the premolars/molars.
- An adhesive bridge attached to the canine alone or the canine plus the central incisor or first premolar.

(b) The ideal choice would depend on the findings of a careful assessment of the possible abutment teeth and the occlusion.
- The canine and central incisor appear to be sound teeth without previous restorations and with good gingival condition. If the lateral incisor had been lost through trauma, the teeth on either side might also have been damaged and should be checked for absence of root fracture or necrotic pulp. If these teeth prove to be sound it would be inadvisable to damage them by preparation for full-coverage crowns, which eliminates the selection of a traditional bridge of fixed–fixed or simple cantilever design.
- If an assessment of the occlusion shows that there is adequate clearance to allow the placement of the wing or wings of an adhesive bridge without interference from the opposing teeth, then the choice would be such a bridge.
- If radiographic examination of the canine reveals a substantial root and occlusal forces are not expected to be severe enough to cause rotation a single wing cantilever adhesive bridge attached to the canine would be the most acceptable and least obtrusive.
- If occlusal forces are expected to be more substantial, a second retentive wing, either on the central incisor or the first premolar, could be contemplated.
- If, for lack of space, an adhesive bridge is precluded, a spring cantilever bridge from a molar or premolar may be considered, the choice of abutment tooth being determined by selection of whichever tooth has already been damaged by a previous restoration.

142 (a) The wear scar is caused by the direct contact with the opposing tooth. Wear at non-contacting sites is caused by the abrasive effect of particles in the diet together with a contribution from toothbrushing.
(b) Wear at the occlusal contact area (OCA) is termed attrition, while wear at the contact-free area (CFA) is termed abrasion.
(c) No. Three terms are use to describe tooth wear. As with materials, the term attrition is used to describe wear at contacting sites; erosion describes the loss of surface resulting from acid dissolution. Abrasion is used to describe any wear which cannot be ascribed to the other two mechanisms. Examples of abrasion are toothbrushing defects, pipe-smoking grooves and hairgrip notches. However, it is generally accepted that more than one mechanism may be involved at any site. The term non-carious loss of tooth substance is becoming more common to describe these combined effects.

143 (a) Large carious cavities are present on the mesial and distal aspects of the upper left central incisor. Access is usually gained from the palatal aspect because this approach usually avoids showing the filling material when the patient smiles.
(b) These lesions are too large to manage by purely preventive procedures. They are well into dentine and cavitated to produce uncleansable plaque traps. Restoration will restore integrity of the tooth surface and aid plaque control. Lesions as large as this may also prejudice pulp vitality and cause pain.
(c) The tooth-coloured filling on the mesial aspect of the upper lateral incisor shows extensive discoloration around the filling, which indicates demineralisation of the underlying

dentine. Since this may represent active caries it would be wise to replace the restoration.
(d) Before a local anaesthetic is given the vitality of the teeth should be checked to ensure that the carious lesion has not progressed to such an extent that the tooth has died.
(e) It is hoped that you do use a topical anaesthetic before giving a local anaesthetic! This is part of careful technique which can make the injection completely painless.

144 The prompt application of a setting calcium hydroxide cement to a small, well-isolated traumatic pulpal exposure may be expected, in most circumstances, to stimulate the formation of a reparative dentine bridge and to preserve the underlying pulpal tissue in a healthy condition.

However, direct pulp capping may not always result in healing of dental pulp and a number of adverse responses may be encountered:

- Physical or microbial insult to the pulp may result in persistent inflammatory changes which may culminate in partial or complete pulpal necrosis.
- Regulation of the mineralisation processes involved in dentine bridge formation may become deranged, resulting in extensive calcification and obliteration of the pulp canal space by mineralised tissue.
- Very rarely, the differentiation of odontoclasts may be induced with the development of internal resorptive lesions.

The possibility of adverse pulpal reactions highlights the need to follow-up teeth which have been subject to pulp-capping procedures.

145 A *cast post and core* is not indicated due to the substantial amount of natural tooth substance that has been preserved. However, some additional retention will be required in order that a satisfactory restoration can be placed. It should also be anticipated that at some time in the future the tooth may require a veneer crown to protect the remaining tissue. This preparation will further reduce core retention.

Additional retention for the core may be gained by placing a *preformed post* in the distal root canal. This canal should be selected in preference to those in the mesial root because it will probably be longer and straighter and therefore less likely to be perforated. The post selected may be of a stainless steel parallel design or a screw post. A post will, however, tend to incorporate stresses in the root as few posts are cemented purely passively. With screw posts there is the additional danger of splitting the root by overtightening.

Retention for an amalgam core may be gained by removing 2 mm of gutta-percha from each root canal, with condensation of amalgam directly into the *open canals*. Although this technique will produce less stress in the root, it will complicate any remedial endodontic therapy.

In addition to packing the canals with amalgam, *slots* may be placed into any available cervical dentine, but it should be recognised that the tooth will be weakened.

Dentine pins may be used in conjunction with an amalgam core but these weaken both the core and the remaining tooth.

An *adhesive core material* such as cermet will gain retention from chemical bonding to dentine and no further tooth preparation for mechanical retention may be required. Unfortunately, the physical properties of this material are inferior to those of amalgam.

146 (a) Following questioning of the patient to discover if the tooth has been traumatised it should be clinically examined. This examination will reveal if the discoloration is related to a break in the external surface of the tooth or to changes within the crown itself. The vitality of the tooth should be determined by the usual means and a periapical radiograph taken so that any alterations in the structure of the crown, root or periapical region may be visualised.

(b)
• Internal resorption.
• External resorption.
• Caries.
• Breakdown products from the blood following trauma.
(c) If the cause of the discoloration is internal resorption, it might be possible to preserve the tooth by undertaking endodontic therapy. For this to be successful, tissue loss must be minimal so that the crown or root is not weakened and the anatomy conducive to preparation and obturation.

External resorption will probably have so weakened the structure of the tooth by the time the discoloration is noticed that preservation is unlikely to be successful.

If the discoloration is due to underlying caries this should be excavated to allow assessment of the size of the cavity in order to determine how best to restore the tooth.

If vital, attempts must be made to prevent trauma to the pulp, producing pulpitic symptoms, while if the tooth is found to have died symptomlessly a decision will need to be taken either to extract or to treat it endodontically. A similar decision will also be required if the discoloration is due to breakdown blood products, although in this instance, if vitality has been preserved and there is no fracture or loss of tissue, no treatment will be necessary.

147 (a) The occlusion is being checked using shimstock. This is 8 μm thick metal foil and if the opposing teeth are in contact, they will hold the shimstock. If the crown holds the foil, but the adjacent natural tooth-to-tooth contact does not, this suggests the crown contact is high. The correct relationship would be when each centric stop/supporting cusp contact holds shimstock.

This assumes that these contacts held shimstock prior to the insertion of the crown and that the patient is not clenching to compress the periodontal ligaments differentially during the procedure.
(b)
• Marginal fit.
• Approximal contacts.
• Shade and morphology.
• Lateral and protrusive excursions.
• Patient satisfaction.
The *marginal fit* should be checked by traversing a probe from the tooth, across the crown margin to the ceramic. A positive edge, where the crown is proud of the tooth surface, is simply corrected by grinding, followed by 'polishing' with diamond paste or, preferably, reglazing. A negative edge is more difficult. Very small discrepancies could be corrected by reducing the tooth margin. Larger defects in the ceramic areas require the addition of low-fusing ceramic and refiring. Defects in the subframe can be corrected by the addition of low-fusing gold solder but there is a danger of cracking the ceramic on cooling after soldering. Anything other than really minor negative edges is best rectified by remaking the crown altogether. The crown should seat onto the finishing line precisely all round the preparation. Any gap would expose cement and be detrimental to the longevity of the crown.

Always check that any error in adaptation is not caused by the *approximal contacts* being tight, thus preventing accurate seating. Check the approximal contacts either by passing dental floss between them or by using articulating paper or a soft pencil to mark the contacting surfaces. A correct contact allows the floss to pass with a click-on gentle pressure.

The *shade* should be checked in natural daylight. If it is too light, then a darker ceramic tint can be fired onto the surface. About half a shade error can be corrected but the difficulty is that the addition of the wash is to the surface only and therefore is not combined into the internal characterisation. It is difficult to lighten a darker shade. Additional firings may affect the ceramic adversely and make the crown appear yellow.

As well as checking the *centric occlusion* contacts, the *excursions* should be checked and adjusted for even contacts using articulating paper. This is particularly important with incisal edge contacts.

The patient should be given the opportunity to see the crowns before cementation. A hand mirror should be held about 2–3 ft (0.7–1 m) away so that the patient sees the appearance as would a casual observer. Holding the mirror very close to the crowns and grimacing into the reflection does not usually show the restorations to their best advantage! If there is any doubt about the patient being happy, then a trial cementation with a weak temporary cement should be undertaken. This allows the patient to receive the reactions of their family and friends prior to a full commitment to the work.

148 (a) Visible light cured, small particle filled composite resin retained by acid-etched enamel.
(b) A careful examination of the right central incisor shows subtle colour differences within the tooth crown. The colour of the central region is dictated by the opacity and shade of the underlying dentine. This tissue extends to within 1.5–2.0 mm of the incisal edge with an irregular border having peaks of colour for each dentine mamelon. The incisal enamel is more translucent than the dentine. Composite resin with different opacity and colour has been applied with careful matching of contour to restore the incisal edge. This restoration matches the contralateral tooth more closely than if a single shade of material had been placed and finished with abrasive discs.
(c)
• Fractured enamel margins are bevelled to expose a large area of cut enamel, which improves bonding and helps the natural colour of the tooth to blend with any slight colour mismatch in the composite resin.
• Teeth become lighter and more opaque as they dry, so shades should be selected before isolating. Most composite resins become darker and more translucent after polymerising and may not match shade guides accurately. A trial restoration can be placed without bonding, before isolating the tooth with rubber dam, to confirm the choice of shades and internal characterisation.
• This is removed, rubber dam applied and the tooth cleaned with pumice and water.
• If dentine exposure is minimal no lining will be required, particularly if it is likely to be visible through the restoration.
• Enamel is acid-etched and the dentine primed before applying an adhesive unfilled resin over the entire preparation surface. A proprietary matrix is placed to support resin lingually, allowing freehand labial contouring.
• Opaque dentine shade resin is shaped and polymerised to replace missing dentine and to form dentine mamelons.
• Enamel shades and translucent resin are added to create a slight overcontour.
• Shaping and development of surface morphology are achieved with tungsten carbide finishing burs.
• Sharp junctions between facets left by the burs are removed with fine abrasive discs and the restoration is polished with alumina paste in a rubber cup to produce a glossy surface.

149 (a) The anhydrous materials comprise a powder which contains the ion-leachable glass and two vacuum-dried acid powders—the poly(alkenoic) acid and tartaric acid. They are mixed with water.
(b) Addition of too much water to a given amount of powder will:
• Reduce the concentration of the polyacid and the tartaric acid for a given quantity of glass.
• Reduce the P:L ratio for that cement in absolute terms.

Both of these alterations will influence the physical properties of the material by extending the working and setting times of the cement, reducing its physical strength and increasing its susceptibility to dissolution in an aqueous environment. Addition of too much water with anhydrous materials is particularly invidious, as the cumulative effects of both reducing the polyacid concentration and alteration in the P:L ratio are greater than the effect of either on their own.

(c) Obviously an encapsulated glass-ionomer (polyalkenoate) cement will have a constant P:L ratio as set by the manufacturer. The mechanical mixing has two additional benefits. The efficiency of the mixing is such that a higher P:L ratio can be used for a given consistency of mix at the end of the mixing process. The encapsulated materials tend to have a fluid consistency, which facilitates clinical handling, but have the same physical characteristics as their hand-mixed counterparts, which are much stiffer in consistency. There is a local heating reaction during the mixing process, which accelerates the setting reaction of an encapsulated product compared with the hand-mixed counterpart.

150 (a) The situation has arisen due to an inadequate embrasure space between the upper first molar and second premolar. The contact point between these teeth has been placed at the gingival margin rather than at the junction between the cervical 2/3 and occlusal 1/3 of the tooth.

(b) Whenever adjacent bridge retainers are fused together it is vital that due consideration be given to the periodontal tissues. Contact points should be established at the correct height and embrasure form designed to allow access by the patient for cleansing. The patient should be given instruction in the use of the correct interdental cleaning aid—e.g. interdental brush, dental floss or tape and threader or Superfloss[17]—to ensure adequate plaque control of this area.

151 Investigations
A history of the symptoms, with a description of the pain, including its location, character (including frequencies and duration), associations and other related symptoms. The pain picture should enable a tentative **diagnosis** to be made. This is likely to include:
• A hyperaemic response to irritated dentine.
• Pulpitis.
• Periodontitis.
Further investigations will be dependent on this tentative diagnosis.
Hyperaemic response
Clinical examination will reveal the presence of exposed dentine and it will be possible to determine whether this is caused by caries, a fractured or lost filling, cervical abrasion or fractured cusp. Sensitivity will be confirmed by probing the area and by the application of heat or cold.
Pulpitis
This is likely to be caused by caries, which may be extensive or recurrent and associated with another restoration in the quadrant. Alternatively, there may be a deep filling with a near exposure or a previous exposure that has not responded to conservative treatment. Since placement of restorations a tooth may have cracked now giving rise to symptoms. Bitewing radiography, vitality tests and the removal of suspicious fillings may all be indicated.
Periodontitis
Teeth may be tender or mobile with or without the loss of supporting bone. Radiographic investigation, periodontal probing and percussion will all be indicated as would examination for the presence of a swelling or the existence of a sinus. Again, vitality testing of suspicious teeth would be appropriate.

Treatment

This would be according to the cause.

Hyperaemia
• Cover dentine with glass-ionomer or amalgam.
• Desensitise dentine with fluoride varnish.

Pulpitis
• Reversible—replace the restoration with a sedative dressing followed by permanent replacement over a sub-base of calcium hydroxide dressing.
• Irreversible—root canal therapy, partial pulpectomy or extract.

Periodontitis
• Apical—root canal therapy, extract.
• Periodontal—scaling, root planing, periodontal surgery, restore contact point.

152 (a) The previous amalgam has been removed, revealing caries of dentine. The present cavity has been cut in enamel only.
(b) The cavity requires extending into dentine throughout its outline and the caries should be explored and removed if possible. Conventional cavities—those which are being cut to excise a lesion as opposed to those which are a combination of exploration, excision and prevention—should be extended into dentine throughout to ensure that the periphery and floors are cleared of caries before restoration. There is a danger of progression of caries along the enamel–dentine junction beneath the restoration as has occurred here.

153 (a) Rochette bridge. This bridge is retained macro-mechanically, with large 'rivets' of composite held in countersunk holes through the metal backing.
(b) The metal may be etched and the restoration retained by means of a fluid, conventional luting composite resin (a Maryland bridge) or the metal may be sandblasted and retained by a chemically adhesive cement.
(c) The advantage of the Rochette design is that it can be removed fairly atraumatically by drilling the composite from the holes and tapping the bridge off. This is an advantage when the bridge has been made as an immediate insertion bridge or when it is part of a splint for mobile teeth which may have to be removed. Its disadvantage is that it is less retentive than the other system shown.
    The advantages and disadvantages of the Maryland (or similar) type of bridge are the converse to those of the Rochette bridge. Additional advantages of the Maryland bridge are that the luting cement is not in contact with the oral fluids, the metal framework can be thinner than the Rochette bridge and it can be used in the posterior part of the mouth more successfully, incorporating previous restorations and other design features. These advantages mean that the Maryland bridge should be used in preference to the Rochette bridge other than in the two circumstances described earlier. If the bridge debonds, however, delay in its recementation may occur because of the need to send it to a commercial laboratory for re-etching or sandblasting.

154 (a) Ethyl chloride.
(b) The possible reasons for the lack of response include:
• Tooth is non-vital. It may already be root-filled.
• Insufficient cold source.
• Pulp extensively sclerosed.
• Presence of a thick insulating base.
• High pain threshold.
• Interruption of sensory supply to the tooth.

155 (a) This condition would normally be described as attrition because the primary cause is rubbing between the lower incisal edges and the palatal surfaces of the opposing teeth. However, the cups in the dentine could not be caused by this action because the dentine in the depth of the cups would not contact the opposing teeth. This effect will have been caused either by acid erosion or by the effect of abrasive particles in the diet.

(b) In this situation composite should be used together with a dentine bonding system. Glass-ionomer (polyalkenoate) is contraindicated because it has inadequate wear resistance and amalgam would look unsightly and be non-retentive.

(c) Composite materials, especially those containing hard quartz particles, may abrade away the opposing tooth surface.

156 (a) This ring is an orthodontic separator. After 48 h there will be a gap between these two teeth of about 2 mm.

(b) The separator has been placed to give the dentist direct visual access to the mesial aspect of the upper first molar. A bitewing radiograph showed a carious lesion just into dentine. The patient (a dental student) wanted to know whether there was a cavity present. This separation allowed an impression to be taken which showed a small break in the enamel surface.

157 (a)

    (i) *Ledermix paste*[18]: a non-setting steroid/antibiotic paste.

    (ii) *Life*[19]: a setting calcium hydroxide cement.

    (iii) *Pulpdent*[20]: a non-setting calcium hydroxide paste.

    (iv) *Kalzinol*[21]: a quick-setting reinforced zinc oxide/eugenol cement.

(b) *Life* is chosen because of its ability to stimulate the formation of a dentine bridge to repair the exposure. A setting material is preferred for general use because of its ease of handling and its ability, when set, to protect the exposed pulp from mechanical trauma during condensation of the subsequent restoration.

(c)

- Steroid/antibiotic preparations are likely to reduce or eliminate symptoms of pulpal pathology by killing invading microorganisms and suppressing local inflammatory response. However, a reparative dentine bridge is unlikely to form and, rather than returning to a healthy state, the pulp is likely to undergo necrosis, often without symptoms.
- Non-setting calcium hydroxide preparations are able to stimulate dentine bridge formation to repair the exposure but do not provide physical protection and are unlikely to remain in place during subsequent restoration of the tooth unless they are overlaid by a rigid pulp cap.
- Zinc oxide/eugenol cements are unlikely to stimulate the formation of a reparative dentine bridge and the irritant effects of the eugenol on the pulp may result in necrosis following a period of pulpitic pain.

158 (a) Clinical procedures will consist of:

- Ensuring that adequate reduction of the tooth has taken place, leaving a labial shoulder width of, ideally, 1.5 mm.
- Extending the preparation slightly more into the gingival crevice on the disto-labial aspect.
- When the temporary crown is constructed and cemented it must be checked for over-extension as this will cause gingival recession and the labial margin of the replacement crown will not be camouflaged when fitted.
- The shade should be chosen with a good natural light source and checked in other lighting conditions. If possible the technician who is going to construct the new crown should be included in shade selection.

In the laboratory:
- Care must be taken to keep the metal substructure as thin as possible to allow an adequate thickness of both opaque and translucent porcelains as this will optimise aesthetics.
- The use of the 'shoulder porcelain' technique may also improve the appearance of the new crown.

(b) A metal–ceramic crown is indicated:
- When it is considered that a substantial amount of force (which would lead to fracture of porcelain) will be exerted upon the crown during function.
- When a porcelain jacket crown has repeatedly fractured.
- If a metal palatal surface is required (to reduce wear on opposing teeth).
- When a chamfer finishing line on the palatal surface is required.
- If the palatal surface requires minimal preparation to retain a retentive crown.

(c) Alternative forms of crown which should be considered suitable are:
- A conventional porcelain jacket crown (PJC). This can provide the most natural appearance but has limited resistance to fracture.
- The McLean/Sced or 'twin foil technique' crown resembles a PJC but retains a tin-plated platinum foil when cemented. This offers aesthetics similar to a PJC but the porcelain chemically bonds to the foil and prevents the propagation of microcracks, thus making the crown more resistant to fracture.

159 (a)
- A developmental anomaly.
- An inadequately reduced fracture.
- A habit.
- An inappropriately designed dental appliance.

(b) Careful questioning of the patient will help determine exactly how long the situation has been in existence and if there has been any associated trauma. Likewise, any contributory habits should be identified at this stage and also the possession of any form of dental appliance.

It would be useful to ascertain the reason why the patient is now seeking treatment if the situation has been present for a period of time. Some idea of the patient's expectations of treatment possibilities may also be of help to the clinician.

A clinical examination will be necessary to determine the general oral status and a radiographic assessment may be indicated, depending on these findings.

An analysis of the occlusion with the aid of models mounted on an adjustable articulator may also be considered prior to the formulation of a suitable treatment plan.

(c) If the cause is determined to be iatrogenic the most likely reason will be that some form of appliance has been constructed and worn, probably to increase the lower face height. In the design, nothing will have been incorporated to prevent over-eruption of the lower incisors. If the appliance was worn in the upper arch there should have been an anterior bite plane or, if made for the lower, the incisal edges required to be covered.

160 (a) The feature is the finishing line, which in this case is a chamfer intended to receive a metal margin. In addition, the probe should be used to check that the finishing line is below the junction of the amalgam core and the dentine.

(b) A clear finishing line is essential for accurate reading of the impression and for the technician to know where to finish the restoration. The finishing line should also be given the shape that is appropriate for the chosen material. The chamfer is used for metal margins, allowing minimal tooth preparation with a positive edge. A shoulder would be used for ceramic and metal–ceramic restorations.

Any finishing line should be based on sound tooth throughout its length to provide a good marginal seal and stability of the crown, independent of any core present. The finishing line must be at least 1 mm below any core/tooth junction to protect that junction from marginal leakage. Also, if the finishing line crosses the core/tooth junction, the resulting interface will consist of three entities—crown, tooth and core—and will be vulnerable to plaque accumulation and breakdown.

161 (a) The bridge retainer has become uncemented, allowing unprotected dentine to be irritated by the ebb and flow of oral fluids and their constituents. Such a situation is a strong encouragement for the development of caries.

(b) The diagnosis can be confirmed by drying the area and then pushing the retainer with a finger or pulling it occlusally with a hand instrument and observing its movement and the exudation of fluid or bubbles around its margins. The pulp of the molar could well be inflamed and confirmation of pulpitis could be obtained by reproducing the typical symptoms with the application of cold to the retainer.

(c) The removal and replacement of the whole bridge would be difficult and may create further problems, particularly with the perforation of the premolar root.

- The loose retainer could be removed by cutting through the pontic close to the premolar retainer. What is left of the bridge might give further service if it is deemed to be sound.
- If the molar has not become carious and its retainer is sound it could be separated from the pontic and recemented. If caries has occurred, a new crown may be required.
- As a long shot it may be possible to repair the cut pontic if it is cut in the middle in a direction slanting upwards and distally. Dovetails could be cut into each severed end of the pontic and these could be filled with amalgam or composite after recementation of the distal segment.

162 (a) A silver cermet glass-ionomer cement has been used to fabricate the entire core of the preparation.

(b) All glass-ionomer (polyalkenoate) cements have a low cohesive tensile strength. While these cements are strong enough to withstand large compressive loads, lateral loading of the crown in this case will result in tensile stress developing around the pins on one side of the core. Tensile failure has occurred, fracturing the core and leaving three pins retained in the tooth.

(c) Glass-ionomer materials should be used only where they are unlikely to be subjected to large tensile stress. They may be used to block out undercuts and fill large voids where natural tooth will bear most of the tensile load if opposing cusps are present. The material should not be built into long unsupported crown preparation cores.

(d) In this case a material with a much higher cohesive tensile strength is required. Amalgam or composite resin would be the first choice. A less conservative, but sometimes more appropriate choice would be to root-fill the tooth and provide a post crown.

163 (a) There is a radiopaque restorative material on the mesial surface of the lateral incisor with a radiolucent area beneath it. The appearance is suggestive of recurrent decay.

(b) A mesial glass-ionomer (polyalkenoate) cement restoration has been placed, then a composite resin surface layer attached to the resin. The restorative grade glass-ionomer was radiolucent and is now visible only as a shadow on radiographs. This procedure results in an appearance of recurrent decay associated with a sound restoration.

(c) If a glass-ionomer cement is to be used as a base beneath composite resin then a radiopaque base material should be used. This can be either chemically set or one of the dual-cure light-activated glass-ionomer materials. The surface of the cement may need some treatment to render it more receptive to bonding with the composite resin.

Chemically activated base materials should be placed in relatively thick layers and should be either etched with phosphoric acid for a short period (15 s) or simply washed during the early stage of their setting reaction. If etching is used then it is essential that the surface of the cement be washed thoroughly prior to application of the composite resin.

Light-activated cements will have an air-inhibited methacrylate layer on their surface which will bond well to composite resin. There is a danger that the composite will be placed over the cement before the chemical phase of the setting reaction is complete when the bond strength of the material to the underlying dentine is weak.

164 (a) The *indications* for porcelain veneers are:
• Coverage of labial surface defects, e.g. hypoplasia of the enamel.
• Masking of discoloured teeth, e.g. tetracycline staining, discoloration following loss of vitality.
• Repair of structural damage, e.g. fractured incisal edges.
• Improvement of tooth contour, e.g. peg-shaped lateral incisors.
• Reduction of spacing in cases when orthodontics would be inappropriate.
(b) *Contraindications* include:
• Severe imbrication of teeth.
• Traumatic occlusal contacts.
• Unfavourable morphology.
• Insufficient tooth structure.
• Insufficient enamel coverage.
(c) The veneers are etched with hydrofluoric acid for a period of 20 min. The application of a silane coupling agent just prior to their placement will also enhance the bond that is achieved. It has been shown that the effectiveness of the coupling agent dramatically reduces in proportion to the length of time since its application.

165 (a) Significant stress build-up and cuspal deflection may occur due to polymerisation shrinkage of a large mass of composite resin in an extensive cavity in a posterior tooth. If the composite resin is bonded to the enamel cavity walls via the acid-etch technique and if the cusp has been undermined and weakened by cavity preparation, cuspal flexure may lead to its fracture.
(b)
• Cuspal deflection and risk of cusp fracture can be reduced by placing the composite resin in small increments and by building up the restoration in a vertical or diagonal layering fashion. This will direct the mass of composite resin to shrink towards the bonded cavity wall rather than towards the centre of the cavity.
• If the cavity outline form of the previous restoration was free from marked undercuts then a composite inlay/onlay restoration could be considered as an alternative. By curing the bulk of the composite mass outside the cavity the risk of cuspal fracture would be significantly reduced if not eliminated entirely.
(c) This tooth had previously been root-filled. The fracture line was acid-etched and a layer of light-curing bond resin was used to seal the fracture. This procedure could still have been employed if the tooth was vital. The patient should be reviewed to assess the need for removal of the restoration and/or fractured cusp with, if necessary, a reassessment of vitality. Thought should be given as to the most suitable long-term restorative treatment option.

166 (a) and (b) There are obviously no correct answers to these questions but clearly it would be more difficult to diagnose this lesion without proper isolation and drying, and even more difficult in a domiciliary situation. The relevance of this latter point is that these are the circumstances in which much epidemiology is done and upon which figures are produced purporting to show the prevalence of caries in populations. Epidemiologists can seldom take radiographs for ethical reasons.

(c) and (d) An experienced clinician would expect to find substantial caries in dentine beneath this lesion. Before the more widespread use of fluoride, particularly in toothpaste, lesions like this would commonly have caved in showing cavitation at a much earlier stage. It appears that the effect of fluoride is to increase the resistance of enamel to collapse in this situation, allowing dentine caries to spread more widely before being detected.

167 (a) The inferior dental nerve block is used to anaesthetise mandibular teeth and is achieved by placing local anaesthetic solution in the region of the mandibular foramen which is situated on the medial aspect of the ramus of the mandible, just inferior to the lingula.

The needle is inserted through the mucosa lateral to the pterygomandibular raphe and it passes through fibres of buccinator and some anterior fibres of the medial pterygoid. It enters the pterygomandibular space and should be advanced until it contacts bone on the medial aspect of the mandibular ramus.

(b) The branches of the facial nerve given off in the parotid gland may be anaesthetised if the tip of the needle pierces the parotid capsule. The result will be a facial nerve palsy which prevents the patient from being able to move the muscles of facial expression on the affected side.

(c) The main concern will be the inability of the patient to close the eyelid and this may lead to desiccation of the cornea or its trauma because of the absence of the blink reflex.

The patient should be reassured that full function will be restored once the anaesthetic solution has dissipated. The eyelid should be taped closed or an eyepatch provided. Preferably a review appointment should be arranged for the following day.

168 (a) (ii)–(iv) inclusive; (i) is incorrect because if the neighbouring tooth is missing wedging will clearly not be feasible and (v) is just not possible.

(b) (iv), (vi) and (vii). If the cavity margins have not been finished and unsupported enamel remains, this may fracture in function leaving a 'ditch' around the amalgam. Similarly, if a 'flash' of amalgam remains at the cavity margin this may fracture, again leaving a ditch. Moisture contamination may cause the restoration to expand and stand proud of the cavity at the periphery. Again, these margins may fracture in function.

(c) (i)–(iii) inclusive. (iv) is incorrect because, while some adjustment of occlusal anatomy can be undertaken at the polishing stage, definitive carving should be undertaken while the material is still plastic. (v) is debatable. Perhaps an attempt could be made to remove minimal areas of porosity but, other than this, other defects of faulty manipulation would necessitate replacement of the restoration. Unfortunately, not all aspects of incorrect manipulation of amalgam will be obvious at an early stage, becoming apparent only with the passage of time.

169 (a) Both upper incisors exhibit crack lines. The left central appears to change colour in the mid-coronal region, with the incisal portion being rather more opaque than the cervical section. There is an ulcer visible on the upper lip.

(b) The trauma sustained by the patient resulted in the fracture of both central incisors. The teeth have been repaired by cementing the tooth fragments together using a dentine–enamel bonding system and a low-viscosity bonding resin. The incisal portion of the left tooth has a greater opacity as it has become desiccated during storage in a paper tissue between the incident and repair.

(c) The complications for these teeth are similar to those for any anterior tooth subject to trauma. They include loss of vitality, progressive pulpal calcification, root resorption and discoloration of the remaining tooth tissue in association with loss of vitality (this would affect only the cervical fragment). In addition, there will be a tendency for the repair line to become more visible as the tooth fragments rehydrate and the resin adhesive absorbs moisture and, possibly, stain from the environment. Subsequent management may include the use of a buccal surface veneer to mask any colour change that occurs within the tooth tissues or the luting resin.

170 (a) The mesio-occlusal restoration in the upper first molar has fractured, leaving an uncleansable plaque trap on the mesial buccal aspect of this restoration. It would be sensible to replace this filling to aid plaque control. Before placing the rubber dam the occlusion should be checked with articulating paper to see whether the occlusal contact in this area has contributed to failure of the restoration. Once the amalgam has been removed, particular care should be taken with this aspect of the restoration to produce a robust amalgam–margin angle.

(b) The restoration in the upper premolar was placed 1 week previously. The filling was left marginally 'high' and occlusal contact has produced this shiny spot. The patient noted some sensitivity for 24 h on biting but the restoration (and tooth) are now comfortable.

(c) The wedge on the mesial surface of the upper molar prevents the dentist cutting the rubber dam with a bur while the cavity is being prepared.

171 (a) Anti-expansion solution.

(b) The addition of *potassium sulphate* (setting accelerator) and *borax* (setting retarder) in the correct proportions allows the control of the setting rate of the plaster. A swiftly setting material is desirable to allow rapid fixation of study casts in the correct relationship to the articulator. This will minimise the risk of articulation errors brought about by the movement of models or articulator components in relation to each other. The addition of a controlled amount of setting retarder allows adequate working time for the necessary manipulation of the material without unduly compromising its rapid setting rate.

Plaster of Paris undergoes expansion during its setting reaction, which may lead to a distortion in the relationship between study cast and articulator. The addition of potassium sulphate and borax reduces the setting expansion of plaster of Paris and minimises the risk of distortion due to setting expansion of the mounting medium.

Alizarin red is a pigment which gives plaster of Paris a pink coloration that allows the mounting plaster to be easily distinguished from the study cast.

172 (a) *Figure 155* shows microleakage around a restoration and permeation of the dentine by a dye.

(b) As dentine is tubular and permeable, the existence of a space around a restoration within a cavity will affect the pulp. Bacteria, which may enter as a result of microleakage, can proliferate in a sheltered environment. The metabolic products of these bacteria then penetrate towards the pulp, leading to sensitivity or recurrent caries. Careful use of restorative materials, especially technique sensitive materials such as dentine bonding systems and composites, will minimise this phenomenon. The use of glass-ionomer (polyalkenoate) based materials under composite restorations will considerably reduce the microleakage associated with this material.

(c) Other techniques which may demonstrate this phenomenon include autoradiography, 'artificial caries', pressure techniques (where dye or air forced into the pulp chamber exudes past the restoration) and electrical conductance. Clinically, sensitivity following placement of a restoration, staining at the restoration margin or recurrent caries can be indicative of microleakage.

173 (a) *Figure 156* shows marked loss of tooth tissue. It is difficult to be precise about the exact cause but there is probably an element of trauma (shown by the darkening of the right lateral incisor), attrition and abrasion in this example.

(b) Before treatment can commence it is necessary to determine the vitality of the involved teeth and their precise occlusal relationship. It would appear that there has been over-eruption of the lower incisors into the space requiring restoration.

Because trauma is implicated in the loss of tooth tissue it is necessary for the teeth to be radiographically examined in case there are undiagnosed root fractures.

In order for adequate retention to be achieved for the final restorations serious thought must be given to electively devitalising the central incisors so that post/cores can be constructed. In view of the lack of inter-occlusal space it may be necessary to construct single-piece crowns with integral posts. This will allow the palatal contours to be of minimal thickness.

174 (a) This lesion has resulted from plaque collecting under the bridge pontic as poor pontic design has prevented or hindered plaque removal from the fitting surface.

(b) Recurrence can be prevented by fitting a new or modified bridge with a pontic that has a narrow bucco-palatal contact with the mucosa and which allows easy access for dental floss. It is important to establish that patients are fully aware of the need for regular flossing. Their introduction to Superfloss[17] or a floss threader should be considered.

175 (a) Abrasion.

(b) These are sites where the abrasive slurry is forced over the restoration surface during mastication.

(c) Overcontouring of a composite restoration can leave feather edges of composite at the cavity margin. These thin edges of material are rapidly abraded, exposing the underlying enamel margin.

(d) At the moment no treatment is necessary. However, the restoration should be monitored as eventually the abrasive process will expose the underlying dentine.

176 (a) A ceramic inlay surrounded by a transparent matrix, with a light-conducting wedge delivering light to the gingival area in the distal proximal region.

(b) The matrix prevents excess resin from filling the proximal space. A dual-cure resin is used to cement the restoration because the deeper parts are not accessible to light-curing. Resin at the margins will not set if it polymerises by chemical initiation alone, as this reaction is highly sensitive to air inhibition. Photoinitiators in the resin are far less sensitive and thus leave only a few microns of unset resin at the surface. The transparent wedge and matrix transmit light into the gingival space to set the resin at the restoration margin.

(c) After removing the matrix the proximal spaces must be seen to be clear of resin. Without a matrix this space would fill with large amounts of resin that are extremely difficult to remove once fully polymerised. Severe periodontal problems will result if they are left. Both failure to light-cure the gingival resin—thus leaving unset material capable of washing out at the margins—or its removal prior to polymerisation could cause a space between the restoration and the preparation to develop. Sensitivity, recurrent caries and long-term pulp damage could all follow.

177 (a) There are four possible explanations for the gingival reaction:
- An overcontoured crown or one with a large overhang on its buccal margin. The crown may have been placed in an endeavour to correct malalignment of the permanent tooth.
- Retention of cement excess within the gingival crevice that should have been removed during cementation.

- Retention of gingival retraction cord within the crevice, either from the impression stage or from being placed during cementation to facilitate tissue retraction and moisture control.
- An allergic reaction to the luting agent concerned.

(b) A careful history from the patient would clarify whether there had been any marked change in the form of the crown as a result of the restoration. A clinical and radiographic examination would also be necessary to identify any marginal overhangs or material excess within the gingival crevice. Finally, patch testing may be necessary if allergy was considered to be a possible aetiological factor. This could be due to the luting agent or possibly to the temporary crown material, depending upon the chronology of the problem.

(c)
- Any excess material should be removed from the gingival crevice and overhanging margins reduced. If the latter is required, this will ultimately necessitate replacement of the crown as it is not possible to reglaze the porcelain; if left unglazed, the porcelain will accumulate more plaque than a glazed porcelain surface.
- If the contour of the crown has been modified significantly and this is thought to be the cause of the problem, the crown should be removed and substituted with a plastic temporary restoration. The morphology of the temporary crown can be modified until the gingival reaction ceases and then a new crown constructed to mimic the modified restoration.
- If an allergy is identified, the crown will have to be removed and recemented with a luting agent to which the subject is not hypersensitive.

178 (a) Diagnosis of failure of any amalgam restoration should commence with a thorough history, clinical examination and radiographic assessment. The failure may be due to:
- Fracture of the restoration, which may be either bulk fracture caused by insufficient depth of the restoration or incorrect occlusal contour or
- Marginal failure that results from incorrect cavo surface angles, leading to marginal ditching.
- Failure of retention due to insufficient undercuts or the failure to place pins when they were required.
- Recurrent caries.
- Periodontal problems, e.g. overhanging margins or inadequate contact points.
- Pulpal problems caused by, for example, careless operative procedures or pre-existing but undiagnosed pulpal pathology.

(b) Marginal fracture of the amalgam has occurred on the buccal cusp due to inadequate carving of the amalgam on placement. This has led to a thin flash of amalgam being left beyond the cavity margin, which has subsequently fractured. Providing there are no signs of recurrent caries, clinically or radiographically, the treatment would be simply to polish the restoration to blend in with the tooth.

179 (a) Not all missing teeth require replacement. There are, however, a number of clinical situations where thought should be given to the possibility of restoring a missing tooth or teeth by the means of either fixed or removal appliances.
Specific indications for this to be undertaken by the means of bridgework include:
- A limited number of edentulous saddles which would not otherwise be more satisfactorily restored with a partial denture.
- The need to prevent the over-eruption of opposing teeth and the drift of teeth neighbouring the edentulous space.
- The presence of suitable abutment teeth—satisfactory crown/root ratio, adequate alveolar support, absence of apical pathology, etc.
- Aesthetics.
- Patient motivation, including time availability.
- Clinical and technical ability.

Some of the *contraindications* are the direct opposite of those previously given. In addition, there are a number that require further consideration:

- Poor oral hygiene.
- High caries rate.
- Multiple spaces in the arch or teeth likely to be lost in the near future.
- Space not detrimental to the maintenance of arch stability or dental health. This may require monitoring over a period of time with the aid of serial study models.
- Unacceptable occlusion.
- Bruxism.

It must be recognised that for the satisfactory provision of a partial denture patients will also need to maintain an acceptable level of oral hygiene and have had the active caries treated. If the clinical and technical skills do not match the demands of the case, bridgework should not be undertaken because a failed bridge is likely to be more detrimental to dental health than a failed partial denture.

(b) Information that will be required to aid the clinician in formulating a treatment plan should be obtained from:

- A clinical examination to ascertain the general state of the mouth, i.e. caries rate, oral hygiene, tooth mobility, length and position of saddles and occlusal relationships.
- Radiographs to identify caries, alveolar bone support, pulp size, presence of unerupted teeth and buried roots, apical status and root morphology.
- Study models—preferably articulated on a semi-adjustable articulator but not mandatory at this stage—to allow the occlusion to be assessed.
- Vitality tests of the potential abutment teeth and any other teeth in the mouth which arouse a suspicion of doubtful vitality. This will allow their prognosis to be determined at the treatment planning stage rather than after a bridge has been commenced which might otherwise have been contraindicated.

180 (a) Gingival irritation caused by food impaction and stagnation as a result of poor contact point formation.

(b) There may be bleeding on probing and hyperplasia of the gingival papillae. If the condition has progressed to periodontitis, a pocket may be present.

(c) There are a number of ways to obtain a good contact with posterior composites:

- Pre-wedging the teeth before commencement of cavity preparation causes minimal displacement of the teeth in the periodontal membrane. Subsequent recovery of this displacement facilitates the formation of a good contact. The technique may cause gingival bleeding when the matrix band is placed and this can compromise the cervical marginal seal.
- Another technique is to wedge a pre-polymerised composite bead between the matrix band and the axial wall of the cavity. If the band is too thin this may result in the formation of a contact nipple rather than a contact point. Also, it is difficult to place the composite around the bead.
- Another method is to use an amalgam condenser to force the composite and matrix band against the approximal tooth while the proximal composite increments are polymerised. This technique should be used with caution because it is easy to bury the tip of the condenser in the polymerised material.

(d) Contact point problems are potentially very serious and need to be treated. Usually the best method is to remove the whole box of one restoration and start again. In this case the contour of the premolar is rather flat, so this would be removed. At that time the contour of the molar could be improved by careful discing.

(e) This is an air bubble in the composite which has been exposed by wear of the restoration surface. The material in the premolar was a two-paste system and air entrapment is a disadvantage of these materials.

181 (a) Metal–ceramic crowns have better aesthetic qualities and will be preferred where appearance is important. Gold is regarded as a more favourable material for occlusal surfaces as its wear characteristics are more in harmony with enamel; porcelain is considered to be the cause of accelerated wear of the opposing dentition. Gold would certainly be preferred for the restoration of occlusal surfaces in the presence of a tooth-grinding habit. The preparation of a full-veneer crown in gold is much more conservative than that for a metal-ceramic crown.
(b) The preparation for a full gold crown involves circumferential and occlusal reduction of between 0.5 and 1 mm to eliminate undercuts and create space for sufficient metal to ensure adequate strength of the crown. In preparing a tooth for a metal–ceramic crown, it is necessary to create space for 0.5 mm of metal plus at least 1 mm of porcelain to ensure adequate strength and optimum aesthetics of the ceramic material.
(c)
• *Full shoulder preparation*—optimum aesthetics with, perhaps, less accurate marginal fit.
• *Shoulderless preparation*—optimum accuracy of fit but a necessity to display metal at the cervical margin which detracts from the aesthetic result.
• *Chamfer preparation and bevelled shoulder preparation*—both represent attempts to achieve better aesthetics than obtainable with the shoulderless style without sacrificing marginal fit to the extent of a full shoulder preparation.

182 (a) Even a well-condensed amalgam that has been placed, carved, burnished and smoothed has a rough surface when examined at a microscopic level. Setting of conventional amalgam produces an initial contractile phase followed by expansion due to crystal growth within the alloy, resulting in a marginally larger (0.04%) amalgam within a 10-h period although this does not necessarily happen with modern alloys. Many alloys do not reach their final dimensions until 24 h after placement. Finishing should therefore be delayed until at least this period has elapsed and should be carried out using a conventional slow speed handpiece.
• The first stage in finishing should be undertaken with stainless steel finishing burs followed by an abrasive impregnated rubber point.
• This is followed by an application of pumice slurry using a bristle brush. The alloy should now be smooth with no obvious excess or deficiency at the tooth–amalgam interface.
• Finally, a rubber cup with zinc oxide powder may be used to produce a high lustre.
At all stages care must be taken to avoid raising the surface temperature significantly, as this can liberate mercury vapour from the restoration or may cause thermal damage to the pulp.
(b) In addition to being able to make small occlusal adjustments, the aim of the procedure is to produce a smooth surface free of pits which may lead to crevice-type corrosion. The margins of the restoration will also be smoothed, decreasing the likelihood of marginal failure. Another benefit of a smoothed restoration is that it will be less plaque-retentive, thus reducing associated gingival inflammation and perhaps recurrent caries.

183
• The upper left central incisor is essentially sound but marred by the discoloured labial composite restoration. This defect is too small to warrant a veneer and the appearance could be improved by simply placing a new composite of the correct shade.
• The upper left lateral incisor is malformed and has had a composite restoration placed which is unsightly. The incisal tip needs to be lengthened. The options are a large composite tip, a ceramic veneer or a ceramic full crown. The resulting composite would be extensive and vulnerable to staining and a crown would involve the removal of much sound tooth. The preferred option is the ceramic veneer.

184 (a) The discoloration may be caused by:
- Recurrent caries (new caries developing around the filling).
- Residual caries (old caries that the dentist has left during cavity preparation).
- Corrosion of the filling material.
- Physical presence of the silver-coloured material shining through the enamel.

(b) This author would replace the filling because it seems probable that active decay is the most likely cause of this appearance. However, other dentists may not agree. There is no 'right' answer here!

185 (a) A custom anterior guidance table.

(b) The purpose of the custom anterior guidance table is to direct the incisal pin of the articulator during simulated lateral and protrusive movements by mimicking the constraint provided by the palatal guidance surfaces of the maxillary labial dentition. The guidance table is moulded in self-curing acrylic resin by the incisive pin of the articulator during movement of articulated casts. These surfaces may be modified by diagnostic waxing to produce any desired alterations in anterior guidance. The resulting table is of assistance in the waxing of palatal contours of restorations to provide the correct anterior guidance.

186 (a) The picture shows a gross example of gingival hyperplasia into a crown retainer. The now-sectioned bridge was retained by crowns on both the canine and first premolar. As the patient incised, the bridge was displaced apically, rotating around the canine, which acted as a fulcrum. The result of this has been to cause failure of the cement lute on the first premolar due to resulting tensile forces. As the bridge was adequately retained by the canine, this failure was not noticed by the patient. Caries has been able to progress unhindered on the first premolar, leading to complete loss of the coronal structure. Gingival tissue has then been able to proliferate into the resulting space between the retainer and the carious tooth.

(b) The premolar should be assessed with regard to its suitability for restoration. Radiographic examination using periapical radiographs will offer information on the extent of caries, morphology of root canals and the presence or absence of periapical pathology. If restoration is considered possible the tooth will require endodontic therapy followed by the placement of a post and core-retained crown. At this stage it is worth considering remaking the bridge using only the canines as abutments. If the tooth is considered unrestorable it should be extracted and a denture provided to replace this and the anterior teeth which had been sectioned from the bridge.

187 (a) The teeth should be dried and carefully examined visually with the aid of a good light. This will help ascertain if there is a chalky appearance to the enamel or a colour change indicative of caries of the underlying dentine.

The suspected fissure should not be forcefully probed as this may initiate a break in an intact surface.

Questioning the patient will help the operator determine how regularly the patient has visited the dentist and also their sugar intake.

Finally, radiographic assessment would confirm clinical findings, help assess the pulpal penetration of the lesion and identify undiagnosed interproximal lesions. The radiographs would allow serial monitoring of the development of this and any other potential lesions which it was considered unnecessary to restore at this stage.

(b)
- Leave.
- Fissure seal.
- Local excision (enamel biopsy) and fissure filling with acid-retained composite.
- Dentine excavation as necessary, with suitable cavity preparation to allow an amalgam or composite restoration to be placed.

154

188 (a) Age, state of health, attitude to dental treatment, personal motivation and standard of oral hygiene are important general considerations. More particular factors are the clinical condition of the teeth, quality of previous restorations, crown size and root length, gingival and periodontal health and the quality of bone support.

(b)
• Periapical radiographs and vitality testing of potential abutment teeth.
• Investigation of existing restorations and the replacement of any which are defective.
• Impressions for study casts and occlusal records to allow detailed occlusal analysis.

(c) The existing partial denture replaces 61|24. The space in the 6| region has reduced considerably due to forward movement of 7| and the position of 75| is now judged to be stable. It was considered that restoration of this space by means of a fixed bridge was not essential, although this is a matter which could be reconsidered at a later date.

The replacement of 1|24 was thought appropriate from a functional and aesthetic point of view. The potential abutment teeth (2|135) have substantial clinical crowns and for this reason it was felt that the right lateral incisor would be adequate, thus avoiding the need to involve the canine as an additional abutment tooth. All four teeth were vital, the canine was unrestored and intact and 2|15 were soundly restored. Apart from mild gingival inflammation associated with prolonged wearing of a tissue-borne acrylic partial denture, the periodontal tissues were healthy and radiographic examination revealed good root length and bone support.

It was felt that construction of a single fixed–fixed restoration could put the abutments at 2|5 at risk of cementation failure and it was therefore decided to restore the dentition by constructing two bridges, a fixed–fixed three-unit bridge using 2|1 as abutments and a compound bridge using |35 as abutments to achieve replacement of |24 with the lateral incisor pontic cantilevered forward from the very substantial canine abutment.

189 (a) The typical sensation from a hyperaemic pulp is a slight or fleeting twinge of pain or discomfort. This is commonly triggered by cold or sweet stimuli. Being a totally pulpal reaction the patient usually has no sense of location and is unable to be certain which tooth in the quadrant is responsible. It may even be thought to be an upper tooth and eventually prove to be a lower one. The discomfort lasts only as long as the stimulus is applied.

(b) A hyperaemic pulp is a response to irritation of dentine and a search must be made to discover some exposed dentine that is accessible to cold and sweet applications, such as carious dentine, dentine exposed by fractured enamel or loss of a filling, dentine exposed by gingival recession or cervical toothbrush abrasion. This latter situation, atypically, may allow patients to be correct about the location as they can induce the discomfort by touching the exposed dentine with a fingernail. Dentine can also be irritated by recent cavity preparation or filling, resulting in a hyperaemic response; thus, any recent filling must be suspect. Confirmation by the operator can be aided with a probe or the application of cold. Alternatively, a bitewing radiograph may reveal a small approximal carious lesion or recurrent caries at the cervical margin of a restoration. There may be several teeth that could be responsible for the discomfort and the final confirmation will often be made as a result of covering or desensitising exposed dentine and recalling the patient to discover if the symptoms have been alleviated.

190 (a) The lower right canine and lower left central incisor are in contact with the palatal surface of the upper abutment teeth, leaving no room for the placement of the retaining wings of the bridge (without disturbing the occlusion).

(b) Composite resin has been added to teeth in the lower arch to develop contact with the upper abutment teeth in the intercuspal position. The upper teeth will have been prepared to give at least 0.5 mm clearance between the opposing teeth. It is possible, during the period between preparation and fitting the bridge, for the teeth to move and this space to be obliterated. It is difficult, if not impossible, to provide successful temporary coverage of the prepared abutments to maintain occlusal relationships in contrast to techniques available for use with conventional bridgework. If the delay between tooth preparation and fitting is to be greater than 7–10 days some form of space maintainer is required.

(c) A small area of enamel at the tips of the opposing lower teeth has been acid-etched and an increment of light-cured composite resin placed to contact the abutments to fill the space created by tooth preparation. At the time of fitting the bridge, the resin is simply removed with small abrasive discs and the enamel surfaces polished. Intercuspal occlusion is checked and interferences in protrusive movements adjusted.

(d) If the abutment teeth move between visits, the relationship between them may alter and prevent accurate fitting of the finished bridge. Loss of space between the opposing teeth will create an occlusal interference. Adjustment of the lower teeth may expose dentine as the enamel is thin in this region. Alternatively, metal may be removed from the retainer wings, weakening them to the point where they could fail.

191 (a) The metal particles are intended to modify the physical properties of the cement, giving greater physical strength and wear resistance to the cement mass. They are thought to act by giving an element of ductility to the surface of the set cement: the particles are exposed on the cement, thus lubricating contacts between opposing restorations/teeth. In addition, there are other benefits in that the aesthetics of such materials are poor; hence, glasses can be used which have intrinsically poor aesthetics but nevertheless have better physical properties or exhibit a better setting reaction than their more aesthetically acceptable counterparts. Finally, the inclusion of heavy metal ions imparts a dense radiopacity to the material.

(b) Gold, silver, tin, aluminium and stainless steel have all been sintered with the glass frit to produce classical cermet glasses. The incorporation of silver–tin alloy from amalgam powder to produce Miracle Mix[22] has also been described and appears to have as many benefits as the directly sintered commercial materials.

(c) The clinical indications of these materials revolve around their altered physical properties and their radiopacity.

- It has been suggested that they can be used as long-term temporary restorations in adults or as a definitive restorative material in the deciduous dentition. However, they retain the inherently brittle nature of all glass-ionomer (polyalkenoate) cements and will fracture if large restorations are exposed to functional loads.
- They form ideal restorative materials for interproximal or buccal root surface caries lesions on molar teeth.
- They can be used as a base material beneath composite resin restorations in posterior teeth, especially when the cement is to be brought out onto the surface of the tooth in the open-sandwich technique.
- Finally, they have a role in modifying contours of crown preparations to eliminate small undercuts. They are insufficiently strong to act as an extensive core material in their own right.

192

- Before trying the crown in the patient's mouth a check should be made to ensure that no damage has occurred to the working model. Particular attention should be paid to the die on which the crown has been made. The crown should be seated on the die and both the marginal adaptatation and contact relationship with adjacent and opposing teeth checked.
- Before removing the temporary crown or fitting the permanent crown it is prudent to place a piece of gauze to protect the patient's airway.

- Having removed the temporary crown and ensured that all temporary cement has been cleared, the crown should be lightly seated. If this is not possible the contact points should be examined with the aid of dental floss. If this cannot be passed between the teeth, the contact points should be marked with thin articulating paper and the crown carefully adjusted using a Busch Silent Wheel[23].
- Once correct contacts have been established, if the crown will still not seat, a careful check of its fit surface should be made. A common technical error is to allow the porcelain to overlap the metal substructure. If this has occurred, it should be removed with a fine bur. The inside of the crown may be painted with rouge dissolved in a solvent. When the solvent evaporates a thin layer of rouge will remain which can be used to highlight any areas of the internal aspect of the crown which are 'binding' on the preparation. These should be carefully adjusted.
- After careful assessment of the marginal fit of the crown, the occlusion should be checked in all excursions of the mandible. Any adjustments made to the crown must be carefully polished. If marked alterations of the porcelain have been required, the crown should be reglazed prior to cementation.

193 (a) A family history. The initial appearance is of hereditary amelogenesis imperfecta. Other conditions which produce generalised staining, such as fluorosis and tetracycline staining, do not produce weakness in the enamel, which has resulted in wear and fractured cusps, as in this case.
(b) There is a large classification of amelogenesis imperfecta but the simplest clinical differentiation is between cases with:
- Poor matrix formation but normal mineralisation, which produces teeth with thin, but sound enamel.
- Normal amounts of matrix and poor mineralisation, which produces normal-shaped teeth where the enamel chips and wears (this is the diagnosis here).
- Combinations of poor matrix formation and poor mineralisation.
(c) In a case as severe as this there is no alternative but to crown all the teeth or to extract them. The dentine is usually normal and conventional crowns can be made, but preferably all the affected enamel should be removed. This means that the crown margins are either subgingival or that extensive crown-lengthening procedures must be carried out. In milder cases it may be possible to use composite and amalgam restorations well into adulthood, deferring the provision of crowns.

194 (a) Accurate reproduction of the marginal detail of crown-and-bridge preparations by elastomeric impressions is facilitated by the apical displacement (or retraction) of the marginal gingiva with retraction cord to allow the impression material to record the tooth surface contour 0.5–1.00 mm cervical to the preparation finish line.
(b) Gingival retraction cords are available in a variety of diameters and degrees of stiffness. Cords may be twisted, braided or knitted and may be supplied impregnated with a chemical or as plain/unmedicated cord. Adrenaline, alum, aluminium or zinc chloride and ferric sulphate are added to promote haemostatic or astringent effects. Adrenaline-impregnated cord is currently the most popular choice with dentists.

195 (a) A spherical particle alloy will set faster than a lathe-cut alloy when amalgamated with mercury and will attain its final mechanical properties more rapidly.
(b) The addition of copper to the alloy, either to form a ternary alloy or a silver–copper alloy admix, reduces the corrosion of the set amalgam because the formation of the tin–mercury phase is reduced or eliminated.
(c) While there is a setting contraction followed by an expansion, the overall result of these two phenomena is a contraction which, for modern materials, is between 2 and 20 μm/cm.

196 (a) A spring cantilever bridge.

(b) The palatal bar has been taken from both retainers, compromising the dental papilla and preventing the patient from exercising adequate interdental cleaning in the area.

(c) Depending on the occlusal relationship beween the upper and lower teeth in the lateral incisor region, thought should be given to providing a resin-bonded bridge of the Maryland design using the central incisor and canine as abutments. The metal substructure should be adequately extended over as much of the palatal surface of these teeth as possible without involvement of the incisal edge of the anterior abutment. This will prevent metal shine-through from distracting from the aesthetics. An interproximal groove on the distal surface of the central and mesial surface of the canine will significantly aid retention.

197 (a) Both restorations are showing evidence of wear and fracture.

(b) Incorrect choice of materials. Although the wear resistance of posterior composites has been improved they should be avoided in restorations where all the occlusal stops are on the restoration (as opposed to shared between the restoration and the remaining tooth). Glass-ionomers (polyalkenoate) have little wear resistance and should be avoided on the occlusal surface of the permanent dentition.

(c) Because of the amount of tooth loss, both teeth should be tested for vitality. If a negative result is obtained, endodontic therapy should be undertaken if an intra-oral radiograph indicates suitable canal morphology. Both teeth will require a core of amalgam or composite suitably retained followed by some form of crown to preserve and protect the remaining tooth substance.

198 (a) The occlusal surface has been sandblasted to produce a matt surface.

(b) Marking of highly polished metal occlusal surfaces during occlusal examination and adjustment may be difficult. The production of a lightly roughened matt surface may assist in the identification of occlusal contacts which appear as shiny burnished areas.

199

- Polysulphide material benefits from an extended working time; this is especially useful when taking an impression of several preparations.
- The tear resistance and surface detail are perfectly adequate for crown and bridgework and although the material is hydrophobic it tolerates moisture within the gingival crevice better than polyvinylsiloxane impression materials.
- As polysulphide sets via a condensation reaction (liberating H_2O), the dimensional stability of this material is less than that of addition-cured materials and the model should be poured within 1 h of recording the impression.

A custom-made acrylic special tray is required and the extra step involved in construction of the tray, long setting time and strong odour associated with polysulphide are often regarded as disadvantages of this impression material.

200 (a) Gingival recession with associated tooth surface loss. The most likely aetiology is erosion, but with a possible contribution from abrasion resulting from faulty tooth brushing technique.

(b) If restored, acid-etched retained composite material would be the most appropriate material to use. However, because of the lack of peripheral enamel, especially cervically, and the presence of dentine on the floor of the cavity an intermediary link, in the form of a glass-ionomer (polyalkenoate) or dentine bonding agent, will be needed to provide additional retention. The most suitable composite for use in this area is a microfilled variety.

Glass-ionomer (Type II) could be used in this situation but is less aesthetic.

(c) The use of a material which bonds to tooth substance for the restoration will eliminate the need for tooth preparation to provide retention. The microfilled materials should be selected because the size of the particles (less than 0.04 μm) incorporated into ground polymer powder improves the polishability. It should be remembered that these materials are inappropriate for use in areas subjected to high stress. They are, however, ideal for placement in areas such as those illustrated.

Both glass-ionomers (Type III) and dentine bonding agents will improve the retention of the final restorative material in situations where there is only limited enamel available to which the composite can bond. Both materials bond to dentine and provide a layer to which composites will adhere. The glass-ionomer requires no surface treatment itself in order to effect the bond and can be externalised cervically. The bonding agent co-polymerises with the composite resin and with either the inorganic (hydroxyapatite) portion of the dentine or the organic portion (collagen).

201 (a) A hole is being cut to receive a dentine pin to provide auxiliary retention for an amalgam restoration.
(b) Dentine pins are required when there is insufficient tooth remaining to retain a plastic restoration. Because they introduce stresses in the dentine their use should be restricted to those areas that really need them. The pin hole should be:
- 1 mm central to the enamel–dentine junction to avoid fracturing the enamel
- 2–3 mm deep to retain the pin adequately
- angled parallel to the external root surface to avoid perforation of the ligament or pulp.

202 (a) Success in pulp capping is recognised by the formation of a complete barrier of calcific repair tissue at the site of pulpal exposure. For this to occur the underlying pulp tissue needs to be vital, uninfected and relatively undamaged and the exposure to be of a minimal size (some authorities would say less than 1 mm in diameter). Thus, favourable factors would be:
- Visual evidence of uninflamed (pink) pulp tissue.
- Absence of copious haemorrhage through the exposure.
- No previous symptoms of pulpitis.
- A small non-carious exposure.
- A clean cavity uncontaminated with saliva.

Pulp capping is a last-resort treatment option and should be considered only if the success of complete pulp extirpation and root filling is regarded as unlikely.
(b) Almost by definition pulp capping is undertaken only following a traumatic exposure during cavity preparation on a healthy symptom-free tooth. Immediately an exposure is suspected, complete isolation, preferably with rubber dam, should be instituted to prevent contamination by saliva. The surrounding dentine should be cleaned by gentle spraying with water and dried. Quick-setting calcium hydroxide should be trickled across the exposure, taking care not to apply pressure to the exposed pulp. When set hard, a temporary dressing should be applied, the situation explained to the patient and a review appointment made. In the absence of symptoms and with the continuing vitality of the tooth, the outer part of the temporary dressing can be removed and a permanent filling placed.
(c) Failure of the treatment would be indicated by symptoms of pulpitis at any time or the lack of vital response after several weeks or months. A dentine bridge can sometimes be observed radiographically, which indicates success, but it is not always possible to detect. Its absence, when other factors are favourable, should not be taken to indicate failure.

203 (a) The lower anterior teeth are carrying all the occlusal load because of the lack of any posterior support. The ceramic teeth of the upper complete denture have become worn, producing a highly abrasive surface which slides over the lower anterior teeth. This continually wears dentine exposed on the worn incisal edges and results in persistent sensitivity.

(b) Reduction in height of the lower anteriors has resulted in loss of vertical dimension. To regain this height it is necessary to crown the teeth, but clinical crown height is minimal. Options here would include porcelain fused to metal, or high-strength all-ceramic crowns. An adhesive luting system would improve retention on the short clinical crowns. Adequate posterior occlusal support is required in the form of a removable partial denture (RPD). The lower crowns should be constructed to accommodate the lower partial denture design such that guide planes, rests and suitable undercuts are provided if a simple RPD is to be made. Alternatively, precision attachments could be used to support the lower denture. To complete the treatment a new upper denture is required.

(c) Because the vertical dimension is being altered, it is important to have a perception of the finished crown height and morphology, particularly as a lower partial denture is to be constructed to fit over the crowns. A laboratory diagnostic wax-up of the final crown contours should be shown to the patient. A flexible vinyl stent can be sucked down over a stone duplicate model of the wax-up and used to construct temporary restorations made to the new vertical dimension. The design for the RPD can be checked on the same model.

204 (a) The cervical part of the cavity margin lies in dentine/cementum and so a conventional composite resin restoration is contraindicated. The cavity could be restored by glass-ionomer (polyalkenoate) alone or with glass-ionomer veneered with composite resin.

(b) *Glass-ionomer* alone provides a simple restoration but does not give as good aesthetics as the glass-ionomer/composite laminate or dentine bonded composite restoration.

The *laminate technique* requires that the composite resin and the glass-ionomer cement are feathered out to meet at the cervical cavosurface margin and this is difficult to achieve precisely. If an opaque glass-ionomer is used with a translucent shade of microfilled composite resin, the aesthetics of the restoration may be impaired by the underlying glass-ionomer cement lining.

Dentine bonded composites are favoured in shallow saucerised cavities (butt joint or box-shaped cavities do not favour adhesion) where there is insufficient depth for an adequate thickness of glass-ionomer cement lining.

205 (a) A radiopaque material extending from the mid portion of the occlusal surface towards the distal proximal surface of the tooth.

(b) A tunnel preparation followed by restoration for the management of interproximal caries.

(c) The tunnel preparation should be used for early carious lesions on the proximal surface of teeth that are judged to be too extensive for a preventive approach but where the occlusal surface of the tooth has not decayed. The advantages of the technique are that the bulk of the residual tooth tissue, including the marginal ridge, is retained intact and thus the strength of the tooth is not impaired as much as with a conventional Class II restoration.

(d) The technique was originally described for use with silicate cements. More recently, it has been adapted for use with glass-ionomer (polyalkenoate) materials, especially the encapsulated forms which can be syringed directly into the cavity. Obviously, a radiopaque material is essential to monitor for recurrent decay. The occlusal surface of the glass-ionomer can be finished with a layer of composite resin if that is deemed desirable.

(e)
- Access into the proximal area can be restricted down the tunnel, which may lead to inadequate clearance of the amelo–dentinal junction.
- It can be difficult to ensure that all of the defect is filled with the restorative agent; any voids may not be demonstrable radiographically and could be potential sites for recurrent decay. Breaches of the proximal wall are inevitable and finishing the periphery is poor. There is the potential for poor adaptation of restorative material to residual tooth substance in this area.

206 (a) The patient has a 'submerging' tooth in the lower second premolar region. This will have occurred due to the lack of development of a permanent successor or possibly the development of the tooth germ in an anatomically incorrect position.
(b) Once the neighbouring teeth have gained their occlusal height the submerged tooth will require careful assessment. If there is only minimal occlusal disharmony, no treatment may be indicated. However, if significant, thought can be given to bonding a restoration to the occlusal surface in order to re-establish the occlusal height of the tooth. This is feasible only if the margins of the occlusal surface are readily accessible to instrumentation; otherwise, there is a danger that the approximal surface of the neighbouring teeth will be damaged during preparation and the placed restoration poorly finished in these areas.

If the tooth has submerged to such an extent that it is locked under the maximum bulbosity of the proximal teeth it will preclude this form of treatment, especially if the adjacent teeth have already started to tilt into the space. In these situations the extraction of the submerging tooth is likely to be indicated, with orthodontic tooth movement to upright tilted teeth if necessary, followed by space maintenance and the provision of a minimal-preparation composite-retained bridge.

207 (a) It is said that this type of labial notch is produced by over-vigorous tooth brushing.
(b) It is highly unlikely that excessive tooth brushing could cause the lingual depression. An alternative hypothesis is that some mechanism, not yet fully understood, is causing decalcification of both labial and lingual surfaces and that the decalcified labial surface is being scrubbed away with a toothbrush, exposing another layer to become decalcified. The tooth brushing is therefore probably a secondary rather than a primary aetiological factor.

208 (a)
- The *addition-cured silicone* impression materials show the greatest stability, with only minimal change after removal from the mouth.
- The *polyether rubbers* show a slight setting contraction, after which they remain stable. They must, however, be stored with care as they have a high ability to absorb water and if this occurs the impression will swell and distort. Direct sunlight also has a detrimental effect on the dimensions of the set material.
- *Polysulphide rubbers* show some dimensional change over the first 24 h, after which they are stable.
- *Condensation silicone rubbers* set by a condensation reaction with the liberation of alcohol. This results in a steady contraction after setting, which can continue for several days. In order to ensure that the impression is a true representation of the preparation(s), it should be poured as soon as possible after it has been made.
(b) Both silicone materials set more rapidly than the polysulphide materials and the setting reaction is accelerated by heat. This can be a problem during summer when the material may be starting to set prior to the final seating of the impression tray and leads, potentially, to a distorted impression.

(c) Polysulphide rubbers show the strongest resistance to tearing but, as a result, impressions can distort when removed from areas where deep undercuts are present.

209 (a) This is attrition, resulting from rubbing between the lower incisal edges and the opposing teeth. In this case there is no hollowing of the exposed dentine.

(b) The patient should be dissuaded from any treatment because there is no decay and the tooth loss is not significant. However, it may be prudent to give patients models of their teeth so that the rate of wear can be monitored at future visits.

(c) Wear should not be regarded as a pathological process. Because patients are keeping their teeth for longer we are now seeing the long-term result of these wear processes in the mouth.

210 (a) The lower first molar contains a filling material that is strongly radiopaque. The material is in fact amalgam but metal inlays and cermets have the same appearance radiographically. The upper first molar is restored with a radiopaque posterior composite. Notice it is less radiopaque than the amalgam filling. The proprietary lining material containing calcium hydroxide is visible beneath the composite because it is more strongly radiopaque.

(b) Posterior filling materials should be radiopaque to facilitate the diagnosis of recurrent caries. Radiolucent filling materials may be confused with demineralisation radiographically.

211 (a) The short clinical crown of the premolar reduces the amount of tooth available for crown retention.

(b) The occlusion and the shape of the underlying preparation.

(c) (i) A post and crown should be fabricated as one unit so that retention is intraradicular as opposed to extracoronal. The crown should consist of a single casting of bonding alloy with a porcelain facing.

(ii) The retention of the restoration will depend upon the amount of tooth tissue remaining under the crown. If a near-parallel preparation can be established, it may be possible to bond a crown to the dentine with a combination of adhesive agents. In addition, the incorporation of grooves in the preparation will increase its retentive capacity. To minimise occlusal reduction this surface should be constructed of gold, and the fitting surface sandblasted to maximise adhesion. At cementation the dentine should be treated with a dentine bonding agent and the crown cemented with a chemically cured composite luting cement.

If the length of the preparation is extremely minimal it could be increased by periodontal surgery. This would involve a flap procedure to remove buccal bone in order to ensure that the crest was at least 1 mm below the new gingival margin.

In extreme cases it may be necessary to devitalise electively the tooth and place a one unit crown as described in (c) (i).

212 (a) During the process of full-veneer crown fabrication, the occlusal morphology of the wax pattern is being developed by the P.K. Thomas wax-additive technique.

(b) This process involves the systematic addition of wax to the occlusal surface of the die to produce cusps, marginal and cusp ridges, triangular ridges and secondary anatomy.

(c) Waxing of the occlusal surface by the wax-additive technique allows the precise place-ment of individual functional components of the crown whose position and articulation may be checked before proceeding to the next stage. Such precise control of occlusal features may be difficult if a conventional wax-carving technique is employed.

213 (a) Enamel microabrasion requires the use of an acid to demineralise the enamel and an abrasive agent. Although orthophosphoric acid can be used, the most commonly employed technique uses a proprietary product which contains hydrochloric acid, pumice, aluminium oxide and synthetic diamond abrasives. In the absence of this product, a slurry of hydrochloric acid (18%) and pumice can be applied to the tooth using a rubber cup in a 10:1 speed-reducing handpiece. The tooth should be rinsed with water for 30 s following microabrasion and then have topical fluoride applied to its surface. Use of a well-sealed rubber dam is mandatory to prevent soft-tissue damage.

(b) Localised mottled enamel areas (e.g. those seen in fluorosis) respond best to this form of treatment.

(c) The technique involves removal of a minimal thickness of enamel. In this case, which shows marked tetracycline staining, the discoloration is present both in the enamel and dentine. Therefore, removal of enamel alone will not help the discoloration and indeed may make it more obvious.

214

- Problems associated with patient management may occur because of medical conditions such as cardiovascular disease, which necessitate care with the choice of anaesthetic agent. Nutritional deficiencies may become apparent and existing medications may require careful monitoring and control. Lack of mobility may make attendance for treatment difficult and also make long treatment sessions inappropriate. Adaption to change is less easily accomplished.

- A reduction in manual dexterity may impair the quality of oral hygiene and this, coupled with a reduction in salivary flow and age changes of the oral mucosa, may cause an increased incidence of periodontal disease, gingival recession, tooth sensitivity and vulnerability to root-surface caries.

- Elderly patients may experience difficulties in the adaptation to prostheses and managing the transition from the natural to the artificial dentition.

- In addition to the specific problems of radicular caries, the increased amount of secondary dentine in the older patient may result in carious lesions becoming more extensive before symptoms develop.

- If endodontic treatment is required, obliteration of the pulp chambers and sclerosis of the root canals may make their location and preparation difficult.

- Surviving tooth substance will become more brittle and if cusps are not to fracture in function they may require coverage with cast restorations for protection.

- Healing of endodontic and periodontal lesions tends to be slower in the elderly because of a reduced reparative capacity.

- Other restorative problems likely to be encountered include cervical abrasion, the consequence of long-standing unrestored tooth loss, deranged occlusions and increasingly severe attritional wear.

- Difficult treatment-planning decisions may arise: whether to adopt simple reparative measures involving the provision of simple prostheses and using 'adhesive'materials such as glass-ionomer (polyalkenoate) cement or composite resins, or to undertake advanced work, including removable or fixed prostheses to restore the occlusion and extensive crown work to restore the appearance. It should, however, be remembered that advanced work will require regular maintenance and with advancing age patients will be unable or unprepared to give the on-going commitment that will be required to maintain good dental health.

215 (a) Acid erosion leading to exposure of dentine.

(b) Diet, usually citrus fruit or juices, would be the main factor, although the effect of this could be enhanced by any developmental defect or by aggressive tooth brushing. A number of patients with this condition have diet fads related to fresh fruit. They also brush their teeth more frequently as part of their behaviour, which accelerates the surface loss. This aetiology would be confirmed in the history and by a diet analysis.

(c) It is essential to change the dietary habits by sympathetic counselling. If the acid erosion were to continue, any restorations placed would be vulnerable to marginal breakdown. Because of the extent of the erosion in this case ceramic veneers are indicated. The placement of these is complicated by the exposed dentine. Very minimal preparations, with no further reduction of dentine, should be performed. It is desirable that the margins of the veneers are on sound enamel to ensure good marginal sealing.

At the cementation stage a dentine bonding agent should be applied to the dentine in addition to normal acid-etching of the surrounding enamel.

216 Information and observations that might lead to the suspicion of non-vitailty of a tooth include:
- History of trauma.
- Symptoms of apical periodontitis.
- Anterior crown discoloration.
- A large carious lesion or restoration.
- An intra- or extra-oral swelling associated with the tooth.
- Radiographic evidence of a widening of periapical ligament space or signs of a periapical abscess or cyst.

217 (a) The interface between the veneer and the tooth has failed, either as a consequence of poor laboratory/clinical technique, or because of excessive functional load with failure at the weakest point in the restoration. The tooth is a lower canine which is likely to be involved in lateral guidance and hence the restoration may come under heavy functional load. However, the veneer has failed at the porcelain–resin interface, which usually has a higher bond strength than the resin–dentine interface which appears to be intact. This would suggest that a failure in bonding technique has occurred.

This may result from:
- Poor etching of the porcelain surface with a lack of micro-mechanical attachment for the resin.
- Inadequate silanisation of the glass surface, causing problems with chemical attachment between the resin and the glass.
- Contamination of the etched silanated surface prior to bonding to the resin reducing the efficacy of the resin–porcelain bond.

(b) The fit surface of the veneer should be roughened by etching with hydrofluoric acid to provide some mechanical retention. It would seem best that this be undertaken in the laboratory, and that the veneer should not be placed back on the stone model after etching.

The etched surface should be coated with a silane coupling agent immediately prior to bonding to the tooth surface. There are two forms of coupling agent available: one-part and two-part. The latter need to be mixed immediately prior to use, but seem to give a better result than the one-part materials.

Surface contamination can result from:
- Die stone from the working cast.
- Saliva.
- Resin from a trial attachment for shade determination.
- Glove powder.

Of these, contamination with die stone is by far the most serious, producing a severe reduction in bond strength. It has proved difficult to cleanse the surface after die stone contamination to eliminate this effect. The remaining contaminants either exert little effect or the effect can be corrected by re-preparing the porcelain surface either with industrial spirit as an organic solvent or by washing with water. The use of acetone as a solvent is to be avoided as this appears simply to disperse a contaminant on the porcelain surface rather than remove it. Silane coupling after surface cleansing then ensures return to maximum bond strength values.

218 (a) The placement of these materials requires considerable care with technique and should preferably be carried out under rubber dam. Particular attention is required to ensure adequate condensation of the materials into the cavity and also that complete polymerisation of the resin takes place. It is frequently difficult to produce a satisfactory occlusal morphology and trimming of the restoration can result in damage to the surrounding tooth tissue. In order to achieve an adequate contact area, it is essential that the tooth is pre-wedged. Alternative techniques to prevent an open contact include loosening the band after placement and polymerisation of the gingival increment or the inclusion of precured portions of material. These are wedged against the axial wall of the cavity and stretch the band to contact the approximal tooth surface.

(b) There is reasonable evidence to show that the larger the restoration the poorer the prognosis for this type of restorative material. Similarly, the absence of cariostatic properties can result in recurrent caries beneath the restoration as a result of a poor or inadequate technique.

(c) Greater success has been achieved with this type of material when it has been used to restore minimal cavities in the anterior regions of the posterior sextants of the mouth. These materials are, of course, aesthetically more acceptable than amalgam and in the premolar region may be considered as an alternative. Their use should be avoided where occlusal forces will be transmitted to the restoration rather than the surrounding tooth substance.

219 (a) There is loss of the upper left central incisor which probably occurred some years previously. The upper left lateral incisor and the upper right central incisor have drifted across the space and the rest of the upper left quadrant has followed.

(b) If the patient wishes the aesthetics improved, there are several options:
• Crowning the lateral incisor.
• Veneering the lateral incisor.
• Orthodontics to open the space and the provision of a bridge to replace the missing central incisor.

Crowning/veneering
To crown the lateral incisor to resemble the missing central is the simplest option but is complicated by the size of the space between the canine and the central which is larger than the opposite central.

A diastema could remain which might be acceptable. The disadvantage is that the gingival margin of the crown would be over-contoured because of the relative disparity between the diameters of the lateral root and new larger crown. This may be acceptable if good oral hygiene is maintained. Because of the size of the space, a crown would be structurally more suitable than a veneer.

Orthodontics
To open the space properly, there will have to be extraction of one tooth in the upper left quadrant and considerable tooth movement in the whole upper arch to retract the upper right central incisor as well as teeth in the left quadrant. On completion of this phase of treatment, a bridge could be provided to replace the missing central. While this would give the best aesthetic result its provision would have to be weighed against maintaining the patient's interest during a

long course of treatment. Clearly there has been little demonstration of interest in the past because no treatment was sought immediately following the loss of the incisor.

On balance, the provision of a crown on the lateral incisor to resemble the missing central is the best option.

220 (a) Erosion produces wear in sites where there is no contact between the upper and lower teeth. In this case the labial and lingual surfaces of several teeth are worn to a degree which could not be the result of attrition. With attrition the upper and lower teeth fit well together and there is an approximately equal amount of wear in the upper and lower teeth. Attrition produces flat wear facets whereas erosion produces cupped incisal edges, as can be seen here in the central incisor teeth and one of the lateral incisors. From *Figure 196* there is therefore sufficient evidence to make the diagnosis that this case is primarily erosion rather than attrition. In fact the patient was a chronic alcoholic and it has now been established that chronic alcoholism leads to an increased rate of erosion.

(b) The treatment options are to accept the situation for the time being, to crown all the teeth, to extract them all or to provide overdentures. With crowns a further decision will need to be made about whether to change the occlusal vertical dimension.

(c) The criteria for choosing between these treatment options are related to the patient, the mouth and the individual teeth.

The patient may be content with the appearance and have no symptoms. Sensitivity, even with this amount of wear, is rare. Even from this occlusal view it is obvious that the labial appearance will already be poor and the patient has tolerated this to the present point. It is unwise to coerce patients into extensive treatment as listed in the other options unless their motivation is very strong.

Dental considerations include whether the condition is progressing, and if so at what pace. Has the aetiology been established and can it be prevented? In this case chronic alcoholism is notoriously difficult for the patient to get under control. The implication is that the tooth wear is likely to progress and so a decision is likely to be needed at some point between the other alternative treatment options. The rate of progress of the tooth wear should be monitored with serial study casts unless it is to be treated immediately.

Individual teeth may give rise to localised problems. In this case the sharp enamel edge on 3⌋ was irritating the patient's lip. This may give rise to soft-tissue lesions and so a simple glass-ionomer (polyalkenoate), composite-layered restoration was placed on the labial surface of this tooth to eliminate this sharp edge and no other treatment was undertaken other than long-term monitoring.

221 (a) This Dentatus-type ARLS articulator is a semi-adjustable non-arcon (non-*ar*ticulated *con*dyle) articulator.

(b)

• *Sagittal condylar guidance.* The adjustable element (condylar track) is located on the mandibular component of the articulator, with the condylar sphere on the maxillary section.

• *Bennett angle.* The condylar pillars can be rotated to vary this angulation, which represents the medial translation of the condyles during lateral excursion.

• *Incisal guidance.* The angulation of the incisal table can be varied to reflect the angulation of the anterior excursive guidance.

(c)

• *A facebow transfer* is required to permit the maxillary cast to be mounted on the upper member of the articulator in the correct relationship to the condylar elements.

- *An occlusal record* in the retruded contact position is necessary so that the lower cast can be correctly related to the upper for mounting on the lower component of the articulator.
- *Occlusal records in protrusion and right and left lateral excursions* are required in order to set the sagittal condylar guidance angles.

222 (a) A fixed–fixed adhesive Rochette bridge.

(b) There is gross calculus at the gingival margin. The bridge should not have been made until the oral hygiene was adequate.

(c) Chemically activated composite cements. Light-cured materials are contraindicated because light cannot penetrate through the metal of the bridge.

(d) The more recent designs of adhesive bridge utilise etched or sandblasted metal wings for adhesion and the thickness of the cement layer has been reduced. The overall adhesion of these bridges is greater than the perforated metal design; but because of the thin cement layer, they are less resistant to torsional forces. In some cases one wing may become debonded, but the bridge remains in place. This may allow rapid caries to develop beneath the debonded retainer. If one end of a perforated metal bridge debonds it is more likely to fall out and this is considered an advantage. Many clinicians now feel that two-unit bridges are preferable to three-unit designs because they do not have the potential for an unrecognised debonded retainer. Another advantage attributed to the perforated metal design is that it is the only bridge which can be cleaned at the chairside and replaced without specialist equipment. This view should be treated with caution because a failure often indicates that the design of the bridge needs to be modified.

223 (a) The mirror on the left is a conventional rear-silvered mirror while that on the right is front-silvered (front-reflecting).

(b) Front-silvered mirrors produce a single image of objects being viewed while rear-silvered mirrors produce a double-imaging effect which duplicates the image of any scratches, markings or surface contamination on the surface of the mirror. Double imaging effects may seriously compromise clear visualisation during exacting operative procedures. However, front-surfaced mirrors are more easily marked and may thus equally impair vision.

224 (a) As the patient has lived in an area with a fluoridated water supply, enamel caries—which has occurred in the fissure system of the first molar—has tended to remineralise. This remineralised tissue is of sufficient strength to resist cavitation despite the progress of the carious process into dentine.

(b)

- The tooth should be investigated for vitality of the pulp. If the tooth is non-vital, a decision must be made whether to extract or endodontically treat the tooth.
- A periapical radiograph will be required to assess the viability of endodontic procedures should they be required.
- If endodontics is possible, the tooth should be rendered caries-free and restored prior to the procedure.
- If vital, the tooth should be anaesthetised and rendered caries-free with caries removal from the ADJ taking priority.
- To prevent bacterial contamination of the dentine or any pulp exposure rubber dam should be placed prior to cutting of the cavity.
- The tooth may then be indirectly or directly pulp capped using a setting $Ca(OH)_2$ material on the near or actual exposure, followed by a structural base prior to restoration.

- If the pulp is traumatically exposed, the tooth should be regularly monitored for vitality following restoration. If endodontic procedures are then required the presence of a restoration will aid rubber dam placement and possibly also the measurement of root-canal lengths.
- If the tooth suffers a carious exposure a decision must be made whether to attempt to save the tooth. If this is possible, and the patient motivated, initial endodontic treatment should be provided and the tooth subsequently restored.

225 (a) These are stained bands between the increments of composite that are caused because each increment has an oxygen-inhibited layer on the surface. Together with contraction forces, this leads to the formation of microspaces between the increments which, eventually, become stained.
(b) It is possible to place a single buccal increment and to fill the space between this increment and the remaining tooth. In this case it is imperative to use a transparent matrix band so that the buccal increment can be cured from the buccal surface. For a restoration of this size it may be better to use an inlay.
(c) Hyperplasia of the gingival papilla.
(d) Poor contact point formation. This is common with this type of restoration because the matrix band tends to be displaced buccally, away from the approximal surface.
(e) As a final restoration this is expecting too much from a composite material. Even if adequate contacts can be achieved, the buccal cusp is likely to wear excessively and will eventually discolour. However, the restoration could be used as a provisional restoration prior to crowning.

REFERENCES

Hansen, E.K., Hansen, B.K., Nielsen, F., Olsen, S. and Lind, K. (1984). Clinical short-term study of marginal integrity of resin restorations. *Scand. J. Dent. Res.*, **92**, 374–9.

Welbury, R.R. and Murray, J.J. (1990). A clinical trial of the glass-ionomer cement-composite resin 'sandwich' technique in Class II cavities in permanent premolar and molar teeth. *Quin. Int.*, **21**, 507–12.

APPENDIX: Materials and Suppliers

[1]Gates Glidden: Produits Dentaires SA, Vevey, Switzerland.

[2]Duralay: Reliance Dental MFG Company, Worth, Illinois 60482, USA.

[3]Palavit G: Heraus Kulzer GmbH, Kulzer Div., PO Box 6393, Wehrheim 1, Germany.

[4]Silicoater: Kulzer GmbH, Dental Div., Philip-Reis-Strasse 8, D-6393 Wehrheim/Ts, Germany.

[5]Comspan: Dentsply Ltd, Hammoor Lane, Addlestone, Weybridge, Surrey KT15 2SE, UK.

[6]Panavia Ex: Cavex Holland BV, PO Box 852, Haarlem, The Netherlands.

[7]Superbond: Sun Medical, Kyoto, Japan.

[8]All-Bond 2: Bisco, Inc., 1500W Thorndale, Itasca, Illinois 60143, USA.

[9]Cerec: Siemens PLC, Windmill Road, Sunbury-on-Thames, Middlesex TW16 7HS, UK.

[10]Tempbond: Kerr UK Ltd, Peterborough, UK.

[11]Opotow Trial Cement: ASIS, Teledyne GETZ, Elk Grove Village, Illinois 60007, USA.

[12]Masserann: Micromega, Prodonta SA, 3 Rue de la Mairie, PO Box CH 1211, Geneva 6, Switzerland.

[13]Epipak: ESPE GmbH, D-8031 Seefeld/Oberbay, Germany.

[14]Nordin: Svedia International, CH-1817 Brent, Montreux, Switzerland.

[15]Dicor: Dentsply Ltd, Coombe Road, Brighton, Sussex BN2 4ER, UK.

[16]Crystal Bond: Chaperlin & Jacobs Ltd, 1 Four Seasons Crescent, Kimpton Road, Sutton, Surrey SM3 9QR, UK.

[17]Superfloss: Oral B Laboratories, Aylesbury, Bucks, UK.

[18]Ledermix: Lederle Laboratories, Gosport, Hampshire, UK.

[19]Life: Kerr UK Ltd, Peterborough, UK.

[20]Pulpdent: Pulpdent Corporation, Watertown, Massachusetts 02272, USA.

[21]Kalzinol: DeTrey Div., Dentsply Ltd, Hammoor Lane, Addlestone, Weybridge, Surrey KT15 2SE, UK.

[22]Miracle Mix: GC Dental Industrial Corporation, 76-1, Hasunuma-cho, Itabashi-ku, Tokyo 174, Japan.

[23]Busch Silent Wheel: Busch & Co. GmbH, Postfach 1152, 5250 Engelskirchen, Germany.

INDEX

Numbers refer to Question and Answer numbers.